Heal
Your Inner

Good Girl

A guide to living an unbound life

NICOLA HUMBER

First published in 2016 by Nicola Humber.

www.NicolaHumber.com

ISBN: 9781849149754

For gran. Who inspired and nurtured my love of books all those years ago.

CONTENTS

FOREWORD

I wanted desperately to be the good girl. I wanted to do all of the right things. I wanted to be 'nice' and lovable. I wanted to be liked and basically, I wanted to be totally inoffensive.

But, inside, I am sharp, shouty and brazen. Inside, I am unapologetically self-assured and no matter how much I've 'tried' to be the good girl, I find myself spilling over my carefully defined edges and showing up in spite of my endless attempts to stick to the 'good girl' plan.

Y'see, I used to believe that if I showed up in the world as who I actually was, no one would love me, I believed that the real me wasn't good enough to love. I wasn't shiny enough, I wasn't professional enough, I wasn't...well, you get the picture, right?
I WASN'T ENOUGH.

Then, when I was 34, both my parents, two aunties, a beautiful friend, one uncle and a cousin died in the space of a year. All the people that I loved the most were gone. All the people who I was trying to be the good girl for were no longer here to validate me.

In amongst the grief, anger, loss, and the complete rollercoaster of emotions that comes from being dealt a hefty side swipe from death in this way, came a voice, from deep down in the depths of my womb:

I am allowed.
I am allowed to create however + whatever I want.
I am allowed to show up in all my messy wholeness.
I am allowed to create a business that feels juicy + nurturing.
I am allowed to break the rules.
I am allowed to do things that make other people uncomfortable.
I am allowed to make choices that piss others off.
I am allowed to write + re-write my story however the f**k I want.

I WISH it hadn't taken everyone I love to die for me to realise this. Which is why if you do nothing else, you NEED to read this book.

Cover to cover.

What Nicola has shared in these pages is deep wisdom and insight for anyone that has ever said 'yes' when they actually meant 'no', for anyone that has an inability to receive because they don't believe they're good enough, for anyone who has ever put the needs of others before herself because she doesn't want to be seen as 'selfish' or 'indulgent'.

I still hear the voice of my inner good girl. Often. She wishes more than anything that I wouldn't speak so loudly about taboo subjects like lady landscapes and menstrual cycles. She hides her face in shame that I'm going to cause trouble. Which is why I'm so grateful that Nicola not only shares her personal story so we all feel a little less alone, but that she also shares usable techniques so that we can keep working with our inner good girl, even when we think we've got it all figured out, because she doesn't go away, not completely.

The good news is, you can make friends with her and you absolutely should because she's sweet and all she really ever wanted, and still wants to do, is take care of you + keep you safe.

Let Nicola, through the pages of this book, be your guide to befriending your inner good girl. To help you thank her, heal her and find ways to hang out together that actually feels good.

But most of all, let this book be your permission slip. Permission to trust that being you - messy, imperfect, not always shiny - is enough.

You were always enough and you will continue to always be enough. Just so you know, 'k?

Big love,

Lisa x

Lisa Lister, author of Code Red: Know Your Flow, Unlock your Monthly Super Powers + Create a Bloody Amazing Life. Period and Love Your Lady Landscape: Trust Your Gut, Care For Down There + Reclaim your Fierce + Feminine SHE Power.
www.thesassyshe.com

INTRODUCTION – A RECOVERING GOOD GIRL

My name is Nicola Humber and I'm a recovering good girl.

There, I've said it! Actually at times over the past few years, I felt that I had completely recovered, only to find my inner good girl surprising me with her presence and holding me back in some new (or familiar) way. And whenever that happened I would think, not this again! Surely I'm done with this by now? But no, there she was, my inner good girl letting me know that whatever I was doing (or trying to do) wasn't quite good enough.

So, what do I mean by the inner good girl?

Well, she's the part of you whose only aim in life is to be 'good'. She shows up in different ways for each one of us and she changes at different times of your life (and also depending on who you are with or what situation you are in).

She can be in-your-face or subtly there in the background. She can be quite enigmatic. On one hand, your inner good girl tells you to keep small and quiet and on the other, she wants you to go faster and be the best. Sometimes she's meek and other times she's striving. She has good intentions, but she's a perfectionist and can be a hard taskmaster.

That's why it can feel so confusing and frustrating to listen to her.

You see, your inner good girl is likely to have received many mixed messages over the years – from parents, siblings, friends, teachers, authority figures and society in general. So, she can be pretty messed-up and confused herself. And she passes those mixed messages on to you, because that's all she knows.

What the heck does 'good' mean anyway?

The reason your inner good girl has picked up these mixed messages is that everyone has their own definition of 'good'. Everyone has their own idea of what being 'good' looks like.

If you look up 'good' in the dictionary, here's the kind of definition you'll see:

> *to be desired or approved of.*
> *having the required qualities; of a high standard.*

You can see that the very definition of good is decided upon externally. It doesn't come from within. Someone else decides whether what you do or say is 'to be desired or approved of'. Someone else decides whether you have the 'required qualities'. But who exactly is giving their approval or deciding on the 'required qualities' here?

Well of course, each of us has their own view of what's desirable, what's acceptable, what's a high standard. And these views can vary widely. So it's no wonder that your inner good girl has got confused. There's simply no way to meet everyone's definition of 'good'. It's impossible.

When I asked my online community the question, 'What does the term "good girl" mean to you?', here are some of the responses I received:

Being kind and generous.

Doing what is expected of you, especially [by] the people around you – e.g. parents, teachers, partner, even kids.

To me the term 'good girl' means not behaving in such a way as to disappoint or annoy someone that I care about. It means keeping my mouth shut when I really want to speak the truth. It means putting someone else's feelings and needs above my own.

Doing what you're told or acting in a way that conforms to what's expected of you, even if it goes against what you'd really like to do.

It's that expectation to do the right thing, be polite, make sure others are happy.

Well-behaved, polite, kind, generous.

It was a term my mother used to let me know I was doing what I was told to do: 'Just do that for Mummy, there's a good girl'. So to achieve any kind of love or recognition I have to be a good girl. I scream inside but years of conditioning mean that I comply and go along, don't rock the boat. I have difficulty even knowing what I really want now as I have subsumed myself for so long.

Doing the 'right thing' by others, society, but not necessarily for myself. This might be doing things that your parents, friends, peers or partner would most approve of.

The social conditioning of others' values. She looks out for others and fulfils their needs more often than her own (puts theirs before hers), she is kind, she does what is asked of her, does her best.

Always working a bit harder and saying, 'Yes' to people when I can.

Being dependable, conscientious, compassionate and always going the 'extra mile'.

Conforming to external notions of what 'good' is as defined by either a society, peer group or other social setting, home/work etc.

Sticking to the rules/norms and doing what you are expected to do.

Someone who always sticks to the rules, never gossips, and doesn't have bad thoughts about people that annoy them.

Essentially being a 'people pleaser'.

Doing right by others, what is expected by others. Putting others' wishes before your own.

Being reliable, playing by the rules, helpful, kind, supportive, not rocking the boat, keeping the peace.

Not making a fuss. Pleasing others so you don't make them feel uncomfortable. Being proper. Conforming.

Impeccably behaved, lovely to look at, organised, tidy, quiet.

Quiet, obedient, compliant, small, no trouble!

From these varied answers, you can see that the term 'good girl' means different things to different people. Some see it as being a positive expression and many as something more restrictive and limiting. There are also some strong themes running through the answers – pleasing others, doing what's expected of you, not 'making a fuss' and sticking to the rules. I'll be exploring these themes in more detail throughout the book.

The truth is in running around and trying to please everyone (which is of course an impossible task), your inner good girl has tied herself up in knots. The good girl messages she's passed on to you can impact on your relationships, your work, your health, your parenting, your bank balance and your wellbeing. They can leave you feeling completely burned out. They can leave you feeling like a crazy person. They can leave you feeling like you're SO not good enough (because nothing is ever good enough for the good girl).

The impact of your inner good girl can be exhausting.

And that's why I felt called to write this book. I want to help you identify where your inner good girl is showing up in your life right now and heal any negative, limiting or restrictive impact she's having on you.

Do you have an inner good girl?

So, how do you know if you have an inner good girl who needs some healing?

If it feels like whatever you do or achieve, it's never enough.

If you feel a vague (or obvious!) sense of dissatisfaction in your life, relationships and work (even though everything looks rosy to the outside world).

If you feel tired of striving – the constant need to do the 'right thing' or be your best.

If you feel shame and guilt about the things you've done in your life that you've labelled as 'bad' (these can be huge life events or seemingly insignificant day-to-day happenings).

If you feel depleted emotionally or energetically right now and you don't know why.

If you have a raging frustration within that you mostly keep hidden, except at times when it erupts like a volcano.

These are all good girl warning signs and this book will help you to move through them.

The aim? To heal your inner good girl and connect with another, more expansive, truly authentic part of you – the part I call your unbound self.

Introducing the unbound self

What do I mean by unbound self?

One definition of unbound is: Not restrained or tied down by bonds.

Your unbound self is the you that you were before you started to receive all of the conflicting messages about how you 'should' be. Your unbound self is the you who is free of what others define as 'good'. Your unbound self is free of those bonds that have tied you down over the years.

Throughout this book we'll be cutting those bonds one by one. I'll be encouraging you to step out of the place of limitation that your inner good girl wants to keep you in and into a place of unbound-ness.

This is where your real dreams lie.

This is where you can feel free.

This is where you let go of the 'shoulds' or 'musts'.

This is where you get to be really YOU.

As you read, I'll give you ways to close the gap between your inner good girl and unbound self.

And why is this important? Well, when you're focused on someone else's definition of 'good', then you can't see what you truly want to be, do and have. When you're focused on being 'good', you can't be great. (And I know that you have greatness inside you, just waiting for you to tap into it.)

So let's get going.

I've written this book in two parts. In the first half, I'll be guiding you to identify and get to know your inner good girl better. You'll be discovering where she came from and allowing her to let go of much of the burden of responsibility she has taken on over the years. You'll also be introduced to your unbound self and begin to connect with her more deeply.

In the second half of the book, I'll be highlighting the different ways your inner good girl can show up and impact on your life. There will be exercises to work through, designed to help you live in a more unbound way in all aspects of your life.

You're free to work through this process at your own pace. You might want to read through the whole book initially and then come back to work through the steps one at a time. That will give you the space you need to process new awarenesses and to do the different exercises that I'll be guiding you through.

To help you get the most out of the book, you'll need the following:

- A JOURNAL OR NOTEBOOK – at various points during the book, I'll be encouraging you to write about any thoughts or feelings that are coming up for you. It will be useful for you to have a journal or notebook especially for the Heal Your Inner Good Girl process. (If you feel resistance to journaling, please know that I often have done too. BUT it's a key way to process your feelings and gain insight. By 'journaling' I don't mean anything lengthy or complicated. It's simply making a few notes which will help you to process your thoughts and feelings. You really don't have to spend long writing – a few minutes will often do.)

- TIME AND SPACE – to benefit from this book, I recommend that you carve out some time to work through the exercises (none of them will take longer than 30 minutes). You'll also need a space where you can be quiet and won't be disturbed.

- SPECIAL MEDITATIONS AND RESOURCES – I've created some unique meditations and other resources to help you move through this healing process. You can access them for free on the link below.

www.nicolahumber.com/heal-your-inner-good-girl-bonuses

A word about potency

Before we get started, a note about the way you choose to work through this book. My recommendation is that you embrace the notion of 'potency' in order to get the most out of this process.

As you can already probably tell, I'm rather partial to a dictionary definition or two, so here's another one for you.

Potency – the power of something to affect the mind or body.

Throughout this book, I'll be talking about how bringing new information about yourself into your awareness helps to create change. It will be a very mindful process. I'll also be asking you to adopt an accepting attitude towards yourself. This process is not about bad-mouthing, punishing, banishing or shaming your inner good girl. It's about getting to know, acknowledge and understand her.

Awareness is always the first step to change. But I invite you to take this to the next level as you read this book and work through the healing process.

I invite you to bring in some potency.

In any kind of personal development work, you have a choice.

1. You can read the book, go to the seminar, work with the practitioner, sit back and wait for change to happen.

   Chance of change: Limited

2. You can read the book, go to the seminar, work with the practitioner, engage in some of the exercises and take a few key points away with you.

   Chance of change: Middling

3. You can read the book, go to the seminar, work with the practitioner, do ALL the exercises (even those you feel resistant to), stay curious throughout and commit to growth.

   Chance of change: Super-high

What I mean by potency is super-charging your experience. Potency is a heightened state. It demands focused attention and energy, and it is *very* worth it.

Your unbound self is a potent being. She knows and accepts herself fully. She has many magical qualities herself and sees the magic in life. Whereas the inner good girl tends to hold back, your unbound self will step forward firmly and surely.

When you choose to focus your attention and energy, you invoke potency, i.e. the power to effect change in your mind, body and circumstances. It's like the difference between a lightbulb and a laser beam. Lightbulbs are helpful – they allow us to see and live more easily. However, laser beams are super-powerful. They make a real difference. They stand out and make an impact.

Throughout this book, I invite you to invoke your potency. Commit to giving this process your focused, laser-beam attention and you can't help but create remarkable, powerful change.

Potency is a choice you make.

So, what does potency look like? In terms of reading this book and working through the inner good girl healing process, potency means:

- Going all in.
- Embracing and dancing with the light and the dark.
- Choosing a friend or group to work through the process with.
- Focused attention (rather than multi-tasking).
- Journaling on whatever comes up.
- Full engagement.
- Keeping a sense of magic.
- Powerful curiosity.
- Acknowledging and working through resistance.
- Choosing to express yourself fully.
- Radical appreciation for whatever you discover.

How does that sound?

Consider how you can allow this experience to be more potent for you. Decide which of my above recommendations you will choose to incorporate.

Here's to creating powerful change!

But, before we move on, let me tell you some more about my personal experience of the inner good girl.

My history of being a 'good girl'

I've been told that I was always a good girl. My dad even says that when I was born, I was the perfect baby – quiet and peaceful. And of course, from that I picked up the idea that being quiet and peaceful equated to being 'good'.

I don't know if I was always good (in fact, I'm damn sure I wasn't!), but once my younger sister, Louise, came along when I was two years old, I slipped into the sensible, older sibling role. I'm pretty certain I wasn't particularly sensible at the age of two (that would be weird!), but certainly the 'good girl' persona started to form.

As we grew up, it feels like our roles were set. I was the quieter, more academic, nose-in-a-book, sensible Nicola. And Louise was the more playful, naughty-little-sister. Of course, neither of us always fitted into these roles, but it's often how we were perceived by our parents, teachers and friends.

Because that's the way it works with the different labels that get attached to us in life – one person might be seen as confident, another as shy, someone else as loud, and some as just trouble! The thing is, though, that once these labels are allocated, it's pretty tricky to shake them off.

These labels become expectations – the people around us expect us to stay in the boxes we've been squeezed into. There's no room for something different, something other.

So, once I was labelled as a 'good girl', it was difficult to let it go. And of course, it felt like it was in my interests to keep hold of my label.

It's interesting that as I write, I see myself as the good girl in relation to my sister. Who we are always happens in relation to others – that's how we show ourselves to the outer world. And at a young age I learned that being quiet, being good (or being seen to be good) earned me praise and rewards.

So I kept doing it. I wanted to maintain my good girl status. (Why wouldn't I?) And I carried that role though school to college, to university, and beyond into the workplace.

Of course I did things that were 'naughty' or risky, but I was generally seen as a good girl. Without me realising, it became a label I was deeply attached to. I was firmly in the good girl box and although it was restrictive, it certainly served the function of keeping me safe. However, when we squeeze ourselves into boxes, it becomes more and more difficult to get out. And I had manipulated myself into such a position.

I was the first person in my family to go to university and when a teacher at my middle school first told my parents that I had the potential to do so, this further embedded my good girl status. When I was deciding what degree to do, I chose a subject that I thought I 'should' be doing, a subject that would be useful – business studies.

Although it was a sensible choice, I could never really get fired up about the subject I was studying for my degree. When I was unhappy during the first year of my course, I turned around and blamed my parents for pushing me into making that choice. This was completely confusing for them, as they had put no pressure whatsoever on me to even do a degree, let alone pushing me towards a particular subject. I was simply responding to an internal pressure to make a 'good' choice and deep down that frustrated me.

Whether I was happy or not, I always did very well in my exams. I passed them all relatively easily. The only thing I failed in my teenage years was my driving test and I was mortified. My mum was shocked to see me coming home crying afterwards; I'm sure it seemed like a huge overreaction to her. But for me it felt like my first taste of failure and it didn't fit with the good-girl persona I had established.

After university I looked for a sensible job and I struggled. I would find a job that seemed to fit the bill, but I would only stick it out for a few weeks or months, as I wanted something more (and just didn't know what that 'more' was). All the time, and out of my awareness, an internal battle was going on between my inner good girl and my unbound self. My inner good girl would say, 'Yes, this is the right job for you Nicola' and my unbound self would be urging me on to do something different.

It took me a few years after leaving university to find a job I was relatively happy in and I settled into a career in financial services. Looking back, it was the friends I made and the social side of my work that kept me in finance for so long. But deep down I always craved more freedom.

My inner good girl had had my life all mapped out from a young age. She visualised me walking through town in a smart coat and hat, working as an accountant (because that seemed like the perfect 'good girl' job to me). So working in finance certainly fitted the bill for my inner good girl.

She had always imagined me living in a big, modern house by the sea, having a New Year's Eve party at the millennium when I would be 29, entertaining my friends and family with my husband and two children. (I can still see this image so clearly.)

And in reality none of this materialised.

ause I knew I wanted something else.

My unbound self craved more. But of course I wasn't sure exactly what that 'more' was.

So I drifted. I would work in a sensible job in finance for a few years, sticking to my good girl plan, and then go off and train as a reflexologist, trying to meet my unbound needs. (I realise that maybe reflexology doesn't sound particularly unbound, but I can assure you it felt pretty freeing after working in financial services for five years.)

Then there would be another internal tussle and my inner good girl would persuade me that I needed to get a 'proper' job again, so back to finance I went. This time for seven years with a nod to my unbound self when I took six months off to go travelling.

But throughout this time, my inner good girl made sure I kept succeeding. I always had a qualification on the go, first to qualify as a financial adviser, and then a more technical investment management exam. And whenever I got another qualification, I didn't let myself enjoy the sense of achievement. I was constantly thinking, 'What next?'

Because this is what your inner good girl does. Her eyes are firmly focused on the next 'thing'. There is always more to achieve. There's no time to celebrate; let's get stuck into the next goal on the list (which never ends).

I could have stayed in finance. I was doing well and was financially very comfortable, but my unbound self was restless. She didn't want me to be stuck in an office for the rest of my life. She was tired of the constraints of the nine-to-five. She called to me, 'Nicola, we could have so much fun if you were in control of your time. Surely you could do something else?'

I listened.

But I wasn't sure how I could create the kind of freedom my unbound self craved. As an initial step I moved to another company. I was head-hunted (which certainly flattered my inner good girl), and thought that this could make me happy – a new role, new colleagues, a new opportunity. But in reality, it was all the same. And I felt even more stifled, pushed down and restricted. I yearned for something else, but I had no idea what.

And then, on a spa break, I attended a talk by a hypnotherapist. To be honest, she seemed to be a completely eccentric older woman, not like any hypnotherapist I've met since, but what she talked about and the demonstration she did sparked something in me.

I had never experienced hypnotherapy before, but during that talk I was struck by the power of the subconscious mind, by the profound difference we could make to our lives and others through the language we chose to use. I came home with the seed of an idea. My unbound self was excited.

Maybe this was what I'd been looking for? Maybe I could retrain as a hypnotherapist?

I started to look into it, researching the courses that were available, and my inner good girl went into overdrive.

'Are you crazy?'

'You can't leave a job after only a few months!'

'What will people think?'

'And hypnotherapy? Everyone will think you're mad!'

But I was so unhappy in my job that I had to do something different. And that was a big enough incentive to allow me to ignore my inner good girl.

I leapt.

Within a few months I had handed in my notice, got a part-time job to pay my way, and started my hypnotherapy training. It had all happened so quickly. Suddenly I was studying again and I had no idea of the amount of personal development I was about to embark upon.

During my hypnotherapy training, I started to look at my inner world, the different aspects of me and the way my past experiences had impacted on me. I learned about the power of visualisation and how we can use metaphor and symbolism to create change. I connected with my inner child.

And I learned the difference between how other people perceived me and my internal experience.

This was a true revelation.

One thing that had often come up in my life was the fact that other people saw me as 'calm'. It's a word that had come up time and time again. And in truth it drove me mad! Others saw me as this calm presence, which I certainly can be, but I knew that a lot of the time there was this turmoil going on inside – anger, fear, excitement, anxiety, despondency, elation, jealousy. All of this was going on internally for me, but no-one could see it. I had disowned those parts of me that I didn't deem 'acceptable'. Because my inner good girl wanted to make sure I kept all of this hidden. She didn't want me to show my full self, because she didn't feel it was safe to do so.

For years I had been keeping it all in, every now and again showing these feelings to those closest to me, usually when I exploded in anger and upset. But during my hypnotherapy and then counselling training I started to show more of myself. And it was such a relief.

That process of revealing different aspects of myself continues. It's never over and that's okay. I wonder if there are parts of you that you keep hidden?

In my work I meet so many women who feel they have to be a certain way, who feel that parts of them are unacceptable or shameful. The number of times a client has shared something with me and then immediately said, 'I know that sounds awful' or 'You must think I'm mad?' And the truth is, what they've been talking about is a completely normal part of being human.

When we deny parts of ourselves, it creates resistance, tension and shame. When we shine a light on all parts of ourselves, we expand, let go and connect with others (and ourselves) more deeply.

That's why I wanted to write this book. Maybe in sharing my own process, I can give you permission to be more you?

The idea of the inner good girl had been bubbling away for me for years, but I had never clearly identified her until recently. After six years of running a successful hypnotherapy and coaching practice, I thought I had the personal development piece nailed. In theory I was living the dream, running my own business, life on my terms, freedom and flexibility, going for my goals. Except when I allowed myself to think about it, I didn't feel like I was living the dream.

My husband would often tell me how proud he was of me, that I had created what I wanted in my life and taken the risk to do something different, but I still felt like I was on a treadmill. I would receive wonderful feedback about the work I did with my clients, my blogs and talks and after a moment of pleasure, it quickly slipped away.

I was doing okay financially, but to be honest, however well I did, it never felt like enough. Why? Because my inner good girl was never going to be satisfied. I told myself I was living life on my terms, I was good at saying 'No' to the things I didn't want to do, but the truth was that I wasn't saying 'No' to my inner good girl.

She was in the driving seat, always pushing for more.

When I started my business, my goal was to replace my corporate income (or a little less), see clients and have more time for myself. But once I got up and running, I started to notice other female entrepreneurs online and my inner good girl began a game of what I call 'comparison-itis'.

Whereas before I would have been happy with making £20,000–£30,000 a year, now I started to desire a six-figure income. Whereas before I would have been happy with a thriving hypnotherapy practice, I started to crave a huge online following.

My inner good girl went wild, coming up with endless ideas about what I could do in my business – write blogs, write a book, create an online course, do events, run a retreat, more public speaking, be an expert, write for magazines, run webinars and telesummits...

Over the past few years, I've done all of these things and to be completely frank a lot of the time it's felt exhausting. Because as soon as I did one thing, something else was waiting for me. My goals became ever bigger.

I was always thinking about my business, never switching off. There was always someone for my inner good girl to keep up with and I never allowed myself to enjoy a settled feeling of satisfaction. Although in theory I was living life the way I wanted, nothing had changed. I was still constantly trying to keep up. And I was so tired.

When I finally realised that my inner good girl was still there, keeping me striving and pushing, I began to see that a lot of the clients I had worked with over the years were experiencing the same. Whether women came to me for help with weight loss, fertility, confidence, anxiety or for help in their businesses, there was always an inner good girl telling them they weren't quite good enough as they were.

That perfectionist voice was always asking for more.

And this is what creates anxiety, fear, depression – the gap between who you are and who your inner good girl feels you should be. When you're listening to your inner good girl you're always going to be in a place of resistance, a place of not enough, a place of wanting and dissatisfaction.

And that's not a happy place to be.

As my realisation grew, I began to see inner good girls all around me. I suspect you have one too if you're reading this book?

The process I outline in this book is going to help you close the gap between your inner good girl and your unbound self. Once you recognise, acknowledge and get to know your inner good girl better, you will begin to understand her intentions. She's not trying to hurt you in any way. She's always trying to do the best for you. But as I mentioned earlier, she's super-confused. So it's no wonder her intentions get muddled.

Here's an example. Even the most inspirational advice can be misinterpreted by your inner good girl. Maybe you have heard this quote from Marianne Williamson before?

Our deepest fear is not that we are inadequate. Our deepest fear is that we are powerful beyond measure. It is our light, not our darkness that most frightens us.

We ask ourselves, 'Who am I to be brilliant, gorgeous, talented, fabulous?' Actually, who are you not to be? You are a child of God.

Your playing small does not serve the world. There is nothing enlightened about shrinking so that other people won't feel insecure around you.

We are all meant to shine, as children do. We were born to make manifest the glory of God that is within us. It's not just in some of us; it's in everyone. And as we let our own light shine, we unconsciously give other people permission to do the same.

As we are liberated from our own fear, our presence automatically liberates others.

Now this is an amazing quote. I absolutely love every word of it. But as I was beginning to write this book, I realised that even a wonderfully expansive quote like this could be misinterpreted by the inner good girl.

The idea of 'playing small' is an interesting one, because it will mean completely different things to different people. When I initially read this quote, although part of me felt uplifted and inspired, I could feel my inner good girl kicking in. She saw this quote as a driver to do more, be more, get busier and set bigger goals. Now all of this is okay (apart from the drive to get busy. Busy-ness is often a distraction), but the intention of my inner good girl was skewed.

She saw this quote as a call to step up and have greater ambition. And there's no problem with that except the intention behind this was that she wanted to be seen to be playing a bigger game. The drive came from a need for external recognition and praise.

And that's the key.

If your driver comes from the external world – needing to be approved of, recognised and praised by others – you're setting yourself up for a lifetime of frustration, dissatisfaction and disappointment. If you want to stop 'playing small' just because you feel you 'should' be playing a bigger game (whatever that means), then you're likely to find it very difficult to step up in a joyful, authentic, truly soulful way.

Because whatever you choose to do with your life, it's the intention that matters. It's your intention that influences whether you feel harassed and pressurised, or expansive and excited. That's why throughout this book I'll be reminding you to check in with your unbound self, to make sure that it's this part of you that's the antennae receiving life's wisdom.

And the more work you do with your inner good girl, the more aligned she'll become with your unbound self. I promise.

Symptoms of an over-active inner good girl

As I've mentioned, your inner good girl can show up in many different ways. She's a complex being! I'll be guiding you through the main ways she can impact you during this process, but here are some of the symptoms you can experience if you have an over-active inner good girl.

Anxiety

Depression

Stress

Inability to relax

Chronic people-pleasing

Constant feeling of dissatisfaction

Financial problems

Inability to know what you want

Physical symptoms around your throat – regular coughs, sore throat etc

Destructive outbursts of anger

Sleep problems

Chronic tiredness

Lack of joy

Lack of energy

Alcohol/drug problems

Weight issues

Lack of motivation, lethargy

If you're experiencing any of the above, then this book is likely to help you. As you move through the process, you will find yourself feeling lighter, more connected, more YOU.

A word about the possible impact of change

Before we get started with Part One, please know that as you read this book and work through the Heal Your Inner Good Girl process, you will be impacted in some way. Much of the impact will be positive, as you get to know and connect with parts of you that have been hidden or neglected, often for years.

However, the process I'm outlining here takes place on many different levels – psychological, emotional, physical, energetic and spiritual. So, you may access previously untapped emotions and forgotten memories that could feel uncomfortable. If you feel this is likely to be the case for you, set your intention to work through this process in a way that feels manageable for you. This book is not intended as a replacement for therapy, so if you feel it might be beneficial for you to work on the issues raised with a therapist, then do so. Get the help you need.

It's also possible that you might feel tired or headachey, particularly after working through the exercises in the first half of this book. Know that this is completely normal and make sure you drink plenty of water, eat healthily and rest more than you usually would. Of course, if symptoms persist, then get them checked out with a doctor.

Also know that as you begin to change, your relationships with those around you may well begin to shift too. The changes you will be experiencing as you work through this book are likely to ripple out into all areas of your life. It's not unusual to find yourself having unexpected arguments or misunderstandings with people close to you during a process such as this. Once again, by making sure you give yourself what you need (lots of self-care, rest and space), you will allow yourself and those around you the chance to integrate the changes you are making more comfortably.

Now I hope that hasn't put you off completely! I simply want to acknowledge the power of this process and reassure you that you are likely to feel different in many ways as you work through this book.

So, let's move on to the first part of the process where I'll be helping you to discover where your inner good girl came from.

PART ONE

STEP ONE – WHERE DOES YOUR INNER GOOD GIRL COME FROM?

As we've talked about already, your inner good girl is the part of you that wants to fit in, do well, play by the rules and please others. She craves positive affirmation from those around her and does everything possible to avoid conflict or 'being told off'.

But where does she come from? How did your inner good girl come into being? This question is important as we're certainly not born with an inner good girl. As babies and young children we don't particularly worry about the impact we have on those around us. We don't think, 'Oh, I'd better not ask to be fed in case I upset Mum.'

Children tend to ask for what they want. Generally, they don't try to second-guess or mind-read those around them. They play and create without inhibitions. Children are very connected to their unbound selves. But at some point the inner good girl starts to develop.

We begin to learn that our parents can be annoyed when we interrupt them to ask for something. We get rewarded for being a 'good girl' and told off for 'making a fuss'. People compliment us on being well-behaved (i.e. quiet) and we get the message that quiet equals good and loud equals bad. Our teachers encourage us to fit in and follow the rules. Over a period of time the inner good girl is formed. That voice in our heads starts to tell us to 'Sit up straight, be quiet, don't play up.'

And this can happen very early on. Even as babies, we can instinctively be aware when our parents or caregivers are upset or irritated and start to modify our behaviour to receive a more positive response. As the inner good girl starts to take hold, we begin to question our desires and natural motivations. We start to make parts of us wrong. We start to dim our lights and quieten our voices.

From my experience, both personally and when working with clients, although the forming of the inner good girl is a gradual process, there will often be a key incident where she's set firmly into your psyche. In one powerful moment your inner good girl takes hold.

This first stage of the process is going to be about discovering what that key experience was for you and beginning to reframe it in a more positive way. This is important because awareness is always the first step to change. The information you gain during this step will put you firmly in a position of power.

> *'Nothing is more exciting and rewarding than the sudden flash of insight that leaves you a changed person...'*
> *Arthur Gordon*

But before we move on to exploring the background of your inner good girl, let me tell you about my key experience as an example.

'Absolute rubbish!'

My inner good girl became firmly established after an incident that happened shortly after I had moved up from infants to middle school, so I guess I was about eight or nine years old.

As I wrote earlier, I had always been a 'good girl'. I did well at school and had loved infants school with its emphasis on creativity and play. The teachers saw me as a good pupil and I had felt very comfortable and secure there. But when

I moved up to middle school, I had to re-establish my identity. The teachers didn't know me or how I had always been known as a good pupil.

I remember one day, early on in my new school, when I was in a class with a stand-in teacher. I'm not sure what subject she was teaching us, but she had given us an exercise to do which involved writing. Again, I don't remember exactly what the exercise involved, but I do remember the experience of writing freely.

We were all there writing away quietly and the words were flowing from my pen. I remember finishing first, pleased with what I had done and taking my work proudly up to the teacher at the front of the class.

I expected her to be pleased. I expected her to say, 'Well done Nicola!' and congratulate me on finishing so quickly. Instead, she stopped the rest of the class and said, 'So, this is why it doesn't pay to rush your work. Nicola has finished first and this is absolute rubbish.'

'Absolute rubbish!' I still remember those scathing words. And the deep, sudden shame I felt. Because I thought I had done well; I was expecting praise. And instead I got told (in front of the whole class) that what I had produced was rubbish.

I was in shock. I remember being sat at my desk and wanting to curl up in a ball. I literally wanted to disappear. I had always done well, been top of the class or thereabouts, and here I was being told off for shoddy work in front of everyone.

In that one moment I learned that I had to be more careful. In that moment I learned that it doesn't pay to be free. In that moment I learned that I had to work harder to be a good girl. I took on the powerful belief that it's not safe to be me, which has impacted on me ever since. That experience taught me to step back, to try and second-guess how someone else would receive me and what I had to offer, to question whether I really was good enough.

Not that I went through my life always harking back to that moment in the classroom. I didn't particularly remember it at all. As a little girl, I shook it off and moved on, distracted by school life.

It was only later during my counselling training, when I was asked to remember a time when I had felt shame, that this experience leapt back into my consciousness. I remembered the physical feeling of shame – hot cheeks, a sick sensation in my stomach and wanting to either shrink or run away (freeze or flee). And as it came back into my awareness, after all those years, I knew that something had changed for me in that moment.

My inner good girl had stepped forward and said, 'Nicola, you really can't wing this any more. You need to be more careful, otherwise you'll be found out again. Don't worry, I'll look after you from now on.' That's the moment when I started to really pay attention to my inner good girl. She had certainly been there before, but the reaction of that teacher brought her right to the forefront of my mind.

And (of course) I realise that the teacher didn't intend to shame me. Maybe she was having a bad day? She didn't know me and to her I was a girl who rushed her work and she believed it wasn't up to scratch. Saying that, she didn't have to call it 'absolute rubbish' in front of the rest of the class, but if we're honest we all say the wrong thing sometimes.

I'm just glad I remembered that experience. Because when you have an idea of the key experience (or experiences) when your inner good girl was formed, you can recognise that when you have those moments of doubt and internal criticism, it's really that little, frightened girl inside of you who's talking. And she just wants to protect you, to keep you safe from the big, bad world (as she sees it).

That's why it's so helpful to identify where your inner good girl comes from. Knowing that her intention is to keep you safe will help you to feel more compassionate towards her, which is a key part of the healing journey.

You may already have an idea of the experience(s) that led to your inner good girl taking hold. It's quite likely that as you've been reading, memories have been coming to mind. If so, that's fantastic. This awareness will stand you in good stead for the healing process you've embarked upon in working through this book.

But if you haven't got any clue of when your inner good girl was formed, or if you feel like you've got a huge muddle of memories which might have impacted on your need to be a good girl, then the easiest way to get clarity is to simply ask your subconscious mind.

This is how I work with my hypnotherapy clients. Rather than consciously trying to figure out which memories are particularly important or where a specific issue stems from, we simply use hypnosis to ask the subconscious mind to guide us.

And this is what I'm going to help you to do throughout this process – using a light trance state to help you create new awareness, connect and work with your inner good girl and unbound self.

Hypnotherapy?

So, this is where I need to explain hypnosis a bit more. If you've never experienced hypnotherapy (or if you've only ever seen stage hypnotists), then you may well be quite apprehensive (or sceptical) about trying it for yourself. I felt exactly the same before I started my hypnotherapy training and many of my clients feel the same when they come to see me for the first time.

So here are some facts about hypnosis:

Hypnosis is a natural and familiar state.

People often think that being in a trance will feel really strange and unfamiliar when, in fact, the opposite is true. We all experience a natural trance state at different times throughout the day.

Have you ever been in a meeting or watching a TV show and realised that you've missed the last couple of minutes as your mind has wandered off?

Have you ever driven somewhere familiar and realised on your arrival that you don't remember the whole journey?

These are both examples of very naturally moving into a trance state where you switch off from the external world and your attention turns inward. When you're in this trance state, you're able to access your subconscious mind more easily.

What do I mean by subconscious mind?

It's the deep part of your mind that stores all of the information you've ever been exposed to. From this information, the subconscious creates habits that are designed to protect you and keep you safe. So, even when you think a decision is coming from your conscious mind, it's the subconscious that's in the driving seat. Through hypnosis we can access and communicate with this deep, powerful part of your mind to bring useful information into your awareness and make changes to old habits and patterns.

You are in control when you're in hypnosis.

Many people worry that hypnotherapy involves someone taking control of their mind and getting them to do things against their will. This idea has been perpetuated by films and TV shows. The truth is that you remain in control during hypnosis. If you need to get up and move during the process, you will be able to do this. And no-one can get you to do something you don't want to do.

Your subconscious mind's role is to protect you and it continues this job throughout any form of hypnosis.

In fact, hypnotherapy is a very collaborative process. When I work with a client, I'm acting as a guide and facilitator, helping them to interact with their subconscious mind in the most useful, transformational way. And this is what I'm going to be helping you to do throughout this process.

Hypnotherapy is a magic pill.

This is most certainly not the case! Even though hypnotherapy can help you to achieve powerful and often fast results, it involves engagement and commitment on your part. Clients sometimes come to me for the first time with the impression that they'll just have to sit back whilst I hypnotise them and all of their problems will be solved.

Er, no.

As I said before, hypnotherapy is very much a collaborative process. To see results, you need to be willing to create change and to work with your therapist. Remember what I said about potency earlier? Saying that, it certainly doesn't have to be a difficult process. In my experience, even challenging issues can be dealt with in a gentle (and even pleasurable) way.

That's certainly my intention for the work you will be doing during this book. The idea is not to banish or punish your inner good girl, or to push her away in favour of your unbound self. This process has been designed to help you connect with and form a healing relationship with these two distinct aspects of you, so you can live your life in a more integrated, authentic way.

I will be guiding you to use self-hypnosis – a relaxed trance state, so you can bring useful information into your awareness, enabling you to make changes and shifts at a subconscious level.

The first exercise using hypnosis will be discovering where your inner good girl comes from. You can read through the instructions below and then access the free MP3 where I will guide you through the process.

Throughout the exercise I invite you to be open to whatever comes up. There's often a temptation to dismiss what your subconscious mind presents to you as insignificant or to think that you're just 'making it up'. Know that whatever comes into your awareness during this exercise is coming to you for a reason. Allow your subconscious mind to guide you.

Be curious.

And enjoy it!

Also, please know that this exercise is purely about gathering information. We will be creating a change in your relationship with your inner good girl later in the process.

'I'm knackered!'

The first time I did an exercise like this, I had just started my hypnotherapy training. I was at home, reading an introductory book about hypnosis and there was a very similar exercise to the one I'm about to share with you. The idea was simply to relax and to ask the question, 'When did I first experience this issue?' At the time I was working on my lack of self-confidence, so I asked the question of my subconscious mind, 'When did I first experience this lack of self-confidence?'

A memory immediately popped into my head.

I was walking home from school on my own, aged about seven (I think), and my dad had walked half-way to meet me. As he reached me, he asked how my day had been and I said, 'I'm knackered!'

It was the first time I had ever used that word. I wasn't even particularly sure what it meant, but I must have heard someone else use it, probably an adult, and thought I would try it out. To me, as a little girl, it seemed like a grown-up word and I felt pretty cool to be using it.

But my dad just started to laugh. He didn't tell me off, he just laughed. It must have been funny for him to hear his little girl use this word that seemed so incongruous. And I remember feeling embarrassed, like I had got something wrong. I didn't receive the response I expected and I certainly didn't feel grown-up, like I had wanted to.

So that was it. That was my memory.

At first, I thought, 'Well that can't be right.'

But it was the first time I had thought of that memory, probably since it happened, so it seemed strange for that particular experience to come to mind. And it made sense. The memory did relate to lacking self-confidence – I had said something to seem more grown-up, received laughter in response and retreated back into my shell – a place I had tended to stay for quite some time afterwards.

I had asked the question of my subconscious and it had very clearly given me an answer, like magic. I was amazed. And I've since experienced this time and time again when working with clients. So during this process, trust that your subconscious will guide and support you.

Exercise – Where does your inner good girl come from?

Take some time to read through these instructions before starting and then come back to the beginning to work through the different steps. Please know that you can't get this wrong – whatever you experience is just the way it's meant to be and whatever comes to mind is coming for a reason.

You can access a free MP3 with a recording of this guided meditation here:

www.nicolahumber.com/heal-your-inner-good-girl-bonuses

Find somewhere quiet, a place where you won't be disturbed for the next few minutes.

Make yourself comfortable, either sitting or lying down.

Take some time to settle, allowing your body to be as comfortable as you can possibly be.

You can imagine that the rest of the day, the rest of the week is dropping away from you, as you gently bring yourself into this moment.

Know, in this moment, that all is well.

Bring your attention to your breath, noticing how it naturally and automatically flows into and out of your body.

Notice how your breath flows without you having to try, without you having to think about it.

Know that your powerful subconscious mind is allowing you to receive exactly what you need in this moment.

Take a deep breath in, gently filling your lungs and breathing right down into your belly.

Then breathe out.

Take two more deep breaths in, right down into your belly.

And as you breathe out, imagine you're letting go of anything you don't need in this moment.

Allow your breath to settle once more and turn your attention inwards.

Just notice any thoughts that come to mind, watching them as if you were an observer.

Allow any thoughts to drift across your mind and gently float away from you.

As your mind settles, silently ask your subconscious mind: 'When did I first learn that I had to be a good girl?'

As you ask this question, notice what comes to mind.

Allow yourself to be aware of any memory that bubbles to the surface.

Be open to whatever comes.

You will find that the memory either comes immediately or maybe it will take a few moments.

You may become aware of it as an image, something you hear, or just a sense of what's there.

If you feel like nothing has come to you, simply imagine what memory would come to mind if you thought about the first time you learned that you had to be a good girl.

Take some time to allow the memory to run through your mind.

If the memory feels upsetting for you, know that you can watch it from a distance as if it was a film playing on a screen. Doing this will help you to feel emotionally detached from the experience.

If it feels okay for you to do so, notice what you can see, hear, smell, taste and feel as you run the memory through your mind.

Silently, ask yourself the question:

'What did I learn here? What did this experience make me believe about myself and the world?'

Notice what comes to mind.

After a few moments, silently send thanks to your subconscious for giving you this information.

Allow yourself to bring your attention back into your body.

Gently stretch your arms and legs, wriggling your fingers and toes.

When you're ready, open your eyes, bringing your attention back to where you are.

When you've finished, take some time to journal on whatever came up for you during the meditation. Write about the memory in as much detail as possible:

Where were you?

How old were you?

Who was with you (if anyone)?

What happened?

How did you feel at the time?

What did you see?

What did you hear?

What did you say (or not say)?

What did you learn here?

What did this experience make you think about yourself?

What did this experience make you think about the world and your place in it?

Take some time to write about what this memory means to you now. How do you feel about it?

How do you feel about the younger you?

Write down anything that comes to mind immediately after this experience. You can even draw a picture that represents what happened and how you feel about it.

The wonderful thing about this kind of work is that you will start to form a healing relationship with your inner good girl. Maybe you've been frustrated or angry with her up until now, but when you realise she's actually a very young part of you, you will start to feel more compassionate towards her.

If you find it difficult to connect with a memory the first time you try, don't worry. This kind of work can take a while to get used to. It can help to listen to the meditation two or three times, over the course of a few days. If a specific memory doesn't come as you listen, know that it can come afterwards – maybe when you're out for a walk, as you're in the shower or as you drift off to sleep at night.

Whenever a memory comes to mind, know that it's coming for a reason and ask yourself the questions I've outlined above.

Even if a specific memory comes easily, you may receive more information during the following hours and days. So keep a journal handy, ready to jot down any notes or insights that come to you.

This is all you have to do for Step One. You are purely gathering information, so set your intention to be in receptive mode and be curious about whatever comes to mind.

STEP TWO – GETTING TO KNOW (AND LOVE) YOUR INNER GOOD GIRL

Now you have an idea of where your inner good girl was formed, it's time to get to know her better. Often there can be a temptation to resist those parts of us, and those qualities, that we don't like. And of course, that's completely natural, but it's this resistance that often leads to discomfort.

By opening up to your inner good girl and getting to know her better, you will naturally start to create a shift and life will begin to flow more easily. I promise! Trust the process, my friend.

So, let's dive in and start with a visualisation to connect with your inner good girl, so you can discover more about her. Again it's best to let go of any expectations for this exercise. Just be open to whatever comes to mind and stay curious throughout.

Don't forget to head over to the link below to download a free MP3 of this visualisation.

www.nicolahumber.com/heal-your-inner-good-girl-bonuses

Exercise – Meeting your inner good girl visualisation

Find somewhere you can be comfortable, a place you know you won't be disturbed for the next few minutes.

Take some time to settle and allow your eyes to gently close.

Imagine that the rest of the day, the rest of the week is dropping away from you and bring your attention to your breath.

Just notice how your breath is flowing into and out of your body.

Take three deep breaths in and out. Breathe right down into your belly and feel a natural release as you breathe out.

Allow your breath to settle once more and just let your mind wander wherever it wants to go.

After a few moments, silently ask your mind to take you to a place where you can connect with your inner good girl, a place where you will both feel completely comfortable, safe and secure.

This might be a place you've been to before, somewhere you would like to go, or maybe somewhere completely imaginary. Just notice which place comes to mind and trust that your powerful subconscious mind is giving you the perfect place to be in this moment.

Take some time to look around and notice what you can see in this place: the colours, shapes and textures.

Notice any particular sounds you can hear, any particular smells, and how you feel to be in this place where you are completely comfortable, safe and secure.

As you get to know this special place, very soon you will realise that your inner good girl is there with you.

As you look around now, you will see her there somewhere.

You can move towards her and as you do, you will notice what she looks like.

Notice how old she is.

What clothes is she wearing?

Is she standing, sitting or reclining?

Is she facing you or turning away?

What is she doing, if anything?

How do you feel about her?

Does she seem welcoming?

Do you have a sense of how she feels about you?

Take in as many details as you can.

Greet her and introduce yourself – let her know you're her adult self and you would like to get to know her better.

Notice her reaction. If she says anything in return, carry on the conversation for a while and see where it leads.

Know that neither of you can get this wrong.

Spend a few more moments together and when you are ready, say goodbye to your inner good girl for now and let her know you'll connect with her again soon.

Gently open your eyes and bring your awareness back to the room where you are.

When you're ready, write about the experience of meeting your inner good girl in your journal. As you do, remember not to judge how this interaction was.

Maybe you already feel loving and compassionate towards your inner good girl?

Maybe you felt angry or frustrated during this exercise?

Maybe you found it hard to connect?

Maybe your inner good girl didn't want to be in your company?

Maybe you found it difficult to be in hers?

Know that it's all okay.

Like I said, neither you nor your inner good girl can get this process wrong.

For now, accept what is and know that this is all part of a healing and integrating journey. There's no need to rush.

When you've finished journaling (and you don't have to spend very long doing this – even five minutes will do. Although, of course, feel free to spend longer if you wish), go and do something completely different. Go for a walk, clean the kitchen, go to the gym, garden – anything that takes you out of your head and into your body for a while. This will allow your subconscious to process what's just happened without your conscious mind questioning it and getting in the way.

You will know when you're ready for the next stage. If you had a fairly positive interaction with your inner good girl, then you can move onto the next exercise fairly quickly. If connecting with her felt more challenging, you may want to take a couple of days before moving on. Give yourself the time you need.

There are two exercises in the next stage and you can choose to do them in whichever order feels good for you. Read through both of them and notice which exercise would feel best to do first. Trust your intuition here.

Exercise – Taking your inner good girl for a walk

I'm a big believer in the healing power of walking. It's my go-to activity if I want to create a shift in my mood and it never fails. There's something about moving in nature that feels inherently good.

So, this is a chance to get outside with your inner good girl and take her for a walk.

When I did the 'meeting your inner good girl' visualisation, I found myself in my childhood bedroom and, to tell you the truth, it felt quite stifling. The room was fine when I was a child, but I've certainly outgrown that space and I immediately felt like I wanted to spend some time with my inner good girl somewhere different.

So, when I had finished journaling, I took her out for a walk (and now I'm inviting you to do the same).

Take some time and go for a walk in a place where you love to go. As you walk, imagine that your inner good girl is there with you.

Maybe she's walking by your side or even sat on your shoulder (this is what happened when I imagined my inner good girl with me).

As you walk, imagine that you're talking with her. Let her know why you're choosing to spend time with her.

Point things out along the way.

Let her know that you appreciate all she's done for you in the past and that now you can maybe both choose to do things differently.

Let her know which things she doesn't have to be responsible for any more – your career, finances and relationships, for example.

Invite her to play.

Just be in her presence.

The idea is that you spend some time with your inner good girl outside and in movement.

The act of doing this can't help but create a shift in your relationship.

Notice how your inner good girl changes throughout the walk. (Of course, this is all imaginary, but when you harness the power of your imagination in this way, just like you did all the time as a child, you create healing and transformation at a deep, subconscious level. And it's fun!)

When I took my inner good girl out for a walk, she started off by sitting on my right shoulder. She seemed a little reticent and guarded at first.

After a while, the conversation started to flow between us. I gave her lots of encouragement and reassurance and before long she was wanting to get down from my shoulder and explore the common where we were walking. When we started the walk home, she got up on both of my shoulders and I carried her down the road. She seemed freer and more joyful.

It was a really lovely experience to spend time with her.

As always, don't set out on your walk with a specific expectation. See what happens and let your interaction flow naturally. You can journal on your experience when you return home.

Exercise – Writing a letter to your inner good girl

The second exercise about getting to know your inner good girl (which you may choose to do before or after the walk) is to write a letter to her.

Writing a letter can be a deeply intimate, cathartic experience. If you felt any anger or frustration towards your inner good girl, this exercise will be particularly beneficial, because you will be able to get a clearer idea of how she feels and her intentions.

Take a sheet of paper and imagine that your inner good girl is writing a letter to you.

I recommend that you write this letter with your non-dominant hand. It will feel awkward, but by doing this you are able to access a different, more creative part of your brain. By using your non-dominant hand, you're less likely to analyse and censor the words that come to you from your inner good girl.

Just put the pen to paper and allow the words to come without judgement or criticism.

What does your inner good girl write?

Let her write whatever she needs to. Know that this letter is likely to be quite short and simple, because she is a child. It's possible that it may only be one or two words. Whatever comes, trust that it's okay.

When her letter has finished, notice how she signs off.

How do you feel to read her words?

Take some time and when you are ready, write a letter back to your inner good girl.

Use this letter to respond to whatever she has written to you. Acknowledge her words.

You can then say anything you need or want to say to your inner good girl. It's your letter, so include whatever feels good for you.

Here are some ideas:

Tell your inner good girl how you feel about her.

Let her know how you've been experiencing her up until now.

Let her know what you appreciate about her.

Ask her what she would like from you.

Ask for what you want from her.

Set some clear boundaries.

Suggest how your relationship could be different.

Send her love.

Draw something for her.

These are just some ideas and remember you're writing to a child, so be mindful of the language you use and keep it simple, so your inner good girl can understand you.

When your letter feels complete (and remember, you can't get any of these exercises wrong), sign it and seal it in an envelope.

Place the envelope somewhere safe and know that your inner good girl has heard what you've said.

Notice how you feel mentally, emotionally, physically and energetically after writing the letter.

Once you have written these initial two letters, you can continue the process of communicating in writing if you choose to.

Allow your inner good girl to write another letter back to you and see what else she has to say.

You can also write another letter to her if that feels good.

Often the initial two letters will be enough, certainly for now, but know that you have the option to write to each other at any time. It can be a great way to hear your inner good girl and for you to communicate with her in a focused way.

Once you have completed both the walk and letter, I encourage you to revisit the initial 'meeting your inner good girl' visualisation.

As you do this, notice what's different.

Maybe your inner good girl will look different?

Is she in the same place?

What's she doing now?

Perhaps you'll find she's more interactive with you?

What kind of things does she say now?

How do you feel differently about her this time?

Before you finish this second visualisation, send love and compassion to your inner good girl. You may choose to give her a hug.

Take some time to journal on your experience afterwards.

This stage of the process is important, as you've been building a more resourceful relationship with your inner good girl, bringing her out into the open and acknowledging her, whilst letting her know more clearly what you would like from her from now on.

STEP THREE – SUPPORTING YOUR INNER GOOD GIRL

Now that you've spent some time with your inner good girl and begun to build a relationship with her, you will find that a level of trust has built up between you.

As your inner good girl has begun to know who you are, it's a good time to step back into that initial event where she was formed and offer her some support. This means revisiting the first exercise where you discovered your key inner good girl experience.

You might be thinking, 'Well what's the point of that? It's in the past and nothing can change what happened back then.' And in a sense you would be right. I don't have a time machine that you can hop into and return to your childhood. But, as you will have realised during the first two steps, this younger part of you – the inner good girl – is still very much with you and impacting your current life.

The memory that you accessed in Step One likely seemed very real to you as you connected with it. The fact that it came into your awareness shows that it is an important experience in your life, one that has impacted on you in a limiting way. At the time, your younger self experienced a challenging situation, one that brought up uncomfortable feelings like fear, shame and confusion. She was made to feel wrong in some way.

And in some ways that young part of you – your inner good girl – has been stuck in that memory ever since. She's been experiencing that fear, shame or confusion ever since that key event and that's why she's been impacting on the way you live your life. She's been trying to keep you safe and protected from what she experienced back then.

She doesn't realise that as the adult you are now, you're much more able to manage those kinds of challenging situations. As the adult you are now, you have far more resources than you had as a young girl. So it's possible to return to that memory and help your younger self to move through it in a resourceful way. In doing this, it's as if you can release your younger self from having to be stuck in that experience. You can free your inner good girl to experience life differently.

To do this, I'm going to invite you to use your imagination. But please don't underestimate the power of this approach.

I was working with a hypnotherapy client a couple of years ago and she remembered a time when her teenage self had been particularly upset. She had taken herself off because she thought nobody understood her, climbed a tree and sat on a branch, feeling alone and hopeless. In hypnosis I guided my client to step back into that memory and comfort her 13-year-old self.

As the session ended, when my client came out of hypnosis, she told me she remembered very well that day when she was upset and sat in the tree. I was amazed as she said that at the time it had felt as if some kind of supportive presence was there with her. For years she had thought that maybe it was an angel, but after this session she realised that it had actually been her adult self returning to comfort her.

How incredible is that? I knew that hypnotherapy was powerful, but this blew me away. And I've since heard other stories like this too.

So, when we imagine ourselves returning to an earlier time and connecting with younger parts of us, it can have a more profound effect than we realise. And this is what I'm going to invite you to do now.

You are going to offer your inner good girl some support, right back where she needs it, in that initial key event where she became firmly set in place.

Note: If the memory that came to you during Step One felt traumatic or particularly uncomfortable for you, know that you can give yourself permission to skip this step. If you feel like returning to the memory would be too much, you may prefer to find a therapist who could help you with this kind of work. Please be mindful of your own mental health and know that this step is not vital to the whole process. You will still benefit from the rest of the book.

Exercise – Supporting your inner good girl

You can access an MP3 which guides you through this exercise on the link below:

www.nicolahumber.com/heal-your-inner-good-girl-bonuses

Find a place where you can make yourself comfortable, somewhere quiet where you won't be disturbed for the next few minutes.

Take some time to settle and gently close your eyes.

Take three deep breaths, in and out. With each one know that you're breathing in relaxation and letting go of anything you don't need in this moment.

Turn your attention inwards, away from the outside world, and simply allow your mind to drift.

As your breathing settles, ask your subconscious mind to show you the memory where your inner good girl was formed.

Just look at the memory initially, as if it were a frame in a film. Notice what's happening, who's there and what your inner good girl is doing, if anything.

Run the film of the memory through in your mind until it reaches the point when whatever formed your inner good girl has just happened.

Know that you can freeze anyone or anything else in the memory if you need to before you step into it, so you can connect with your inner good girl without being disturbed.

Once you have done this (if you need to), step into the memory and introduce yourself to your inner good girl.

Let her know that you've come back to help her.

Ask her how she's feeling.

Ask her what's just happened.

Be gentle with her.

It may take her a while to feel comfortable with you.

Reassure and comfort her, just like you would do for any child in a similar situation.

Acknowledge how she's feeling.

Let her know that whatever's happened, she's okay. You're there to support her.

Ask her what she would like to do. Perhaps she would like to leave this situation or have someone else she knows and trusts come and be there with her?

Maybe she wants to say something to someone else who's there, to express herself?

Help her to do whatever she needs to in order to feel more comfortable.

Remember, you're the adult and you can use your resources to support your inner good girl now.

Keep reassuring her throughout.

Allow yourself to be guided by your younger self. She will let you know what she wants or needs, so give her the space to do this.

It's important to stay in your adult self. If you feel that you're becoming one with your inner good girl, step back out of the memory and come back into your adult self, before stepping back in.

Once you have helped your inner good girl to do whatever she needs to do to feel better, let her know that she's done really well.

Make sure she feels safe wherever she is now and let her know that you're always here to support her if she needs you.

Say goodbye in whichever way you choose and when you're ready step back out of the memory.

Take a few moments of relaxation.

Gently begin to stretch and move your body and whenever you're ready, open your eyes.

Notice how you feel.

Give yourself some time to journal on how that exercise was for you.

In my experience with this kind of work, it really needs very little guidance. Between you and your younger self, you will be able to figure out what needs to happen.

Once you've made some notes about how the experience was for you, take a break and do something completely different. Get something to eat, have a drink, go for a walk, get out in the garden, take a nap. Allow your body to receive what it needs as your subconscious mind processes the work you've just done.

STEP FOUR – YOUR UNBOUND SELF

Now that you have got to know your inner good girl better, it's time to connect with another part of you – your unbound self. This is the part of you that represents the limitless possibilities that were available to you when you were born. Each of us is filled with unbound potential when we enter the world, but throughout our lives we are told that we have to follow particular rules and ways of being. We're told (either directly or indirectly) that we have to fall in with the 'normal' way of doing things. We learn to fit in, to adapt ourselves to please others, to be a good girl.

But within each of us there is an unbound self, that part of us that is unique, authentic and truly YOU.

'If you ask me what I have come to do, it is this: to live out loud.'
Emile Zola

You will already be more connected with this part of you after working through the first three steps of this process. Now it's time to get to know your unbound self even better, so you can express more of this part of you.

I wonder what your unbound self is like? Let's begin to find out.

Exercise – What does 'unbound' mean to you?

First of all, I invite you to explore what the word 'unbound' means to you. If you were truly unbound, if you let go of limitations, what would that look like?

Take some time to journal on this and write down some ideas. At the beginning of 2015, I did a similar exercise and came up with the following:

I express my truth freely.

I let go of what no longer serves me, limiting beliefs, structures and patterns.

I dance.

I allow my hair to go grey and embrace the wise, wild woman within.

I reach out.

I live in tune with my feminine cycle.

I meet my needs.

I allow myself to receive without limitation.

I choose.

I feel the wind against my skin.

I walk barefoot.

I embrace what is.

I shine my light fully.

I made this into an image, combining the text with a photo of me walking along the beach. A friend commented that I looked like a rock star in the image, and that really represents what unbound-ness means to me!

I still love looking at it and reading the words now. They lift me up.

So I invite you to create something similar now. What does unbound mean to you?

Side-note: Actually, as I re-read the words, I realise I could have been more specific. There are some statements (such as 'I allow my hair to go grey') that are defined actions which I've been able to incorporate into my life, whereas others (such as 'I choose') are more general. Both are okay and the more general statements can certainly feel expansive and freeing, but make sure you have a combination of specific and general meanings.

Once you've done this exercise, it's time to meet your unbound self. Again during this visualisation, keep an open mind to whatever comes up. Allow your subconscious mind to guide you.

As always, you can access a free MP3 of this visualisation on the link below:

www.nicolahumber.com/heal-your-inner-good-girl-bonuses

Exercise – Meeting your unbound self

Find somewhere quiet, somewhere you know you won't be disturbed.

Make yourself as comfortable as you can be and allow your eyes to gently close.

Let your breathing settle.

Bring your attention into your body and notice how you feel physically.

Bring yourself into this present moment.

Imagine that you're breathing in a sense of relaxation, calm and peacefulness, as if with each breath in you're becoming more and more relaxed.

As you enjoy this calm and peaceful feeling, allow your mind to drift, almost as if your mind is floating.

Silently ask your subconscious mind to guide you to a place where you will be able to meet and connect with your unbound self.

Notice which place comes to mind and allow yourself to be there now.

See what you can see.

Hear what you can hear.

Smell what you can smell.

Taste what you can taste.

Feel what you can feel.

As you're there, very soon you will find that you notice your unbound self.

You will sense that she's there with you.

Notice how she comes into your awareness.

Maybe you see her, or hear her, or something else?

Notice how you experience your unbound self.

If you see her, notice what she looks like.

What is she wearing?

How old is she?

Where is she and what is she doing?

Is she moving or still?

Is she sitting, standing or reclining?

How does she relate to you, if at all?

Does she have anything to say to you?

Is there anything you'd like to say to her?

What happens?

Take your time and allow yourself to do, say and be whatever you want.

How do you feel to be in her company?

Does she remind you of anyone?

Spend a few more moments there with your unbound self. Know that you have created a connection that will continue to evolve.

When you're ready, say goodbye to your unbound self for now and gently bring your awareness back to where you are. Stretch and move your body as you open your eyes.

When you have completed the visualisation, take some time to journal about how this experience was for you.

What was it like to meet your unbound self?

What did you learn?

How do you feel now?

Allow your words to flow and when you've done this, go and do something completely different. This will enable your subconscious mind to process the experience in the best way possible for you.

Be aware that this first meeting with your unbound self might feel quite uncomfortable. Many of us have become so familiar with living in accordance with our inner good girls that coming into contact with a more unbound expression of us feels like a *huge* step out of our comfort zones. Whereas your inner good girl is safe, likes routines and plans, your unbound self is likely to be more wild, unpredictable and ever-changing.

It's possible you may question why you would want to become more acquainted with this wild, seemingly out-of-control part of yourself! I completely understand this.

Although a huge part of the personal development work I've done over the years has involved connecting with and learning to express different parts of myself, when I did the unbound self visualisation for the first time, I felt quite overwhelmed. My inner good girl had been easy to define and make contact with. I could relate to her easily and I felt in control of the interaction.

But my unbound self was a completely different story.

We met on a wild, windy beach and I couldn't make her out at first. She was like a ball of energy and I would get glimpses of a woman with long, tangled hair, the wind and rain lashing her cheeks, but then she would change again. And she wouldn't stop moving. In the end I asked her, 'How can I connect with you if I can't pin you down? You're not solid!' As I read that back, I realise that of course she wouldn't want to be pinned down. She's unbound!

But as I asked she whispered in my ear, 'Don't worry. I'm always here.'

There was something uneasy but exhilarating about the interaction and I feel excited as I write that.

Whatever your initial experience with your unbound self was like, know that the idea is not necessarily to ditch your inner good girl and become 100% unbound. There will always be a spectrum along which you can move freely. Some days you may be more 'good' (whatever that means to you) and other days more 'unbound' (again, whatever that means to you). This healing process has been designed to allow you to access a fuller expression of yourself, to give you more of a choice about how you relate to others and live your life.

The idea is that you're moving towards 'wholeness'. Simply raising your awareness of the different aspects of you, in the way you're doing as you work through this book, will help immensely with that.

So I wonder what would happen if your unbound self and inner good girl were to meet? I wonder how they would interact with each other? I wonder how your unbound self would impact your inner good girl?

Let's find out.

The gorgeous thing about this work is that anything is possible. By harnessing the power of your imagination, you can access forgotten parts of yourself and create powerful awakenings.

Before you begin this next exercise, simply intend for this meeting to be beneficial and supportive. Intention is a powerful tool and we want to ensure that this first interaction between your inner good girl and unbound self is expansive and uplifting.

Head to the link below to access a free MP3 which will guide you through this exercise.

www.nicolahumber.com/heal-your-inner-good-girl-bonuses

Exercise – The meeting of your unbound self and inner good girl

As before, find somewhere peaceful, a place you won't be disturbed.

Make yourself comfortable and gently close your eyes.

Imagine the rest of the day, the rest of the week, is dropping away from you as you bring yourself into this moment.

Know that all is well.

Bring your attention into your body and notice how you feel physically.

Allow a sense of relaxation and calm to flow through you.

Take three deep breaths in and out.

With each exhalation, you can find yourself more deeply relaxed.

As you enjoy this feeling of peacefulness, imagine that there's a large white screen in front of you.

You can choose to see this large, white screen in your mind's eye, just in front of you at a comfortable distance.

As you watch the screen, I'd like you to imagine that your inner good girl and unbound self appear there.

You can see them both appearing on the screen now in whichever way they choose to.

Notice how they look on the screen.

Where does each of them appear on the screen?

What size are they in relation to each other? Is one bigger than the other, or are they the same size?

How do they relate to each other (if at all)?

Do they face each other, stand side-by-side, back to back or something else?

How do you feel as you see both of them on the screen?

Are you more drawn to one or the other?

Know that you can take this time to make any changes you would like to make in the way they appear now.

Experiment with changing their positions or sizes. Notice how you feel as you make any changes.

Ask each of them if they have anything they would like to say to each other.

Hear what they say and notice what this interaction is like.

What does the unbound self want to share with your inner good girl?

How does your inner good girl react to this?

Know that you can facilitate any interaction if you feel it's necessary. You can offer guidance or reassurance if needed.

Take your time with this exercise.

Allow both your unbound self and inner good girl to say and do whatever they need to. When this feels complete for now, thank them both.

Allow the screen to become clear and notice how it feels to have that space.

Bring your attention back into your body. Gently stretch and move, before opening your eyes and bringing your awareness back to the room where you are.

Notice how you feel after the interaction. As always, take some time to journal on the experience. Write about the interaction between your inner good girl and your unbound self in the present tense, for example, 'I see my inner good girl in the left-hand corner of the screen', rather than 'I saw'. This will help you to feel more present in the experience as you write about it.

Be aware that these are two very different parts of you, so the interaction may be uncomfortable, unbalanced, confrontational or unsettling. However the experience is for you, know that it's okay.

As I've said before, this is a transformational process and change often feels challenging.

As you've been working through the exercises in this book, you're been creating shifts in your psychological, emotional and energetic bodies and this is not to be underestimated. As I mentioned at the beginning of the book, it's possible that you may feel tired, under the weather, have headaches or muscular aches, feel emotional or extra sensitive after doing these exercises. All of that is completely normal. You are expanding. You are growing. You are healing old patterns and creating new pathways. So it's important that you look after yourself as you move through this process. Rest, eat well, spend time in nature and ask for support if you feel you need it.

Well done for working through Part One of this process. You truly have come a long way.

Now it's time to move on to Part Two…

PART TWO

So, where does your inner good girl show up? I wonder if anything in my own story of being a 'good girl' resonated with you? Maybe the need to constantly push and strive or not appreciating the moment is something you recognise in yourself?

Or perhaps there's a part of you that yearns for more playfulness, excitement and adventure in your life and your inner good girl is keeping you 'on track' (and by on track, I mean the inner good girl's idea of the right track)?

In this second half of the book, I want to help you notice where your inner good girl is showing up in your life right now. How is she impacting on you? Before any change comes awareness, so if you want to connect with your unbound self at a deeper level, then this step is key.

But this part of the process may not be completely straightforward, as the inner good girl is very enigmatic. She doesn't show up in the same way for everybody. In fact, she can show up in very different ways for the same person at different times.

She is a conundrum.

And that's why she had me confused for years.

I didn't realise that the same part of me that sometimes wanted me to keep quiet and be overly polite was the same part that urged me on to host big events or try and create a six-figure business. I couldn't see how the same part that wanted me to colour between the lines when I was little was the same part that was also constantly pushing me to move outside my comfort zone.

And I really couldn't fathom how the same part of me that would say 'Sorry' if there was any inkling that I'd done something wrong was the very same part that wanted me to be forever achieving more.

You see, your inner good girl is as wonderfully complex as you are. And that's what can make her hard to pin down (and completely frustrating at times!).

So, pinpointing how she shows up in your life can be challenging. But in the following chapters, I'm going to be sharing some of the areas of life I've noticed the inner good girl making an appearance for myself and my clients over the years.

STEP FIVE – GOOD GIRL GOALS

I have a love–hate relationship with goals. As a coach and hypnotherapist I know they're important to create clarity, focus and motivation. But they can also feel like a pressure and you can end up feeling like a failure if you don't achieve the goals you set for yourself.

So how can you set goals that inspire you rather than make you feel like crap? The key thing is not to be duped into setting good girl goals.

Good girl goals

What the heck do I mean by good girl goals? Good girl goals are goals that you feel (or rather your inner good girl feels) you should be achieving.

Recently I was working through a personal development exercise in a book I was reading and I had to write down a list of goals that would stretch me. I actually felt quite resistant to doing this exercise, but when I finally came to do it, I noticed that most of the goals on my list were good girl goals.

How did I know? Well, as I looked at them I felt deflated. I knew that achieving them would be a chore and even if I achieved them, I couldn't really see how they would add much to my life (apart from the fact I could say I had achieved them).

Hint: The inner good girl loves achievement for achievement's sake.

There were a couple of goals on the list that felt different though. I felt excited when I looked at them. I wanted to get going with them straight away. The thought of achieving them felt rich and joyful. These were unbound self goals.

Unbound self goals are super-compelling. They draw you towards them like a magnet. It's as if you can't help but achieve them once you get started (one way or another). Good girl goals always feel like hard work. It's a struggle to reach them and you're left feeling flat when you do (anti-climax ahoy!).

I've seen this time and time again with clients over the years. If someone comes to me with a good girl goal (i.e. something they feel they *should* be doing or something they want to do to please someone else), no matter how much work we do, they struggle to reach it. In fact, when I help them to explore what they *really* want, they often end up tapping into an unbound self goal and creating something completely different in their lives.

Let me give you an example. When I started my hypnotherapy practice, I specialised in helping clients with weight loss. And I found that very often when a client came to me for help with weight loss, there was a good girl goal lurking.

Often my clients would have a particular weight they wanted to get to, but in reality this was just an arbitrary number. On its own it was meaningless and it was difficult to get excited about a number (that's a key reason why so many people struggle with their weight).

I very quickly realised that my clients never wanted to be a particular weight because of the number. This was a good girl goal, driven by 'shoulds' and 'musts' and the external pressure of glossy magazines and advertisements. When we delved deeper, there was always some other reason for wanting to lose weight and this was usually about how they wanted to feel.

Whenever I started working with a new client, I would ask how reaching her weight loss goal would make her feel. Then the answers always started to flow – more confident, energised, sexy, free, healthy, strong.

This was the true unbound self goal. It's the feeling that they were aiming for, not the number on the scales.

Danielle Laporte has written the most wonderful book about this, *The Desire Map*. In it she guides you through a process to discover your Core Desired Feelings and to set goals based on these feelings. If you haven't read it already, I highly recommend getting yourself a copy. (You can find a reading list of recommended books at the back of the book.)

It's always the feeling that will motivate you. The same applies to any other goals you may set yourself.

Now I specialise in helping women with their money mindset, and financial goals have many similarities with weight loss goals. It's easy to pick a number out of the air and say, 'I want to earn that', but it's difficult to be motivated purely by a number.

I've certainly found this over the years in my business. At times I've often struggled with reaching financial goals. Whenever I've reflected on this, I've found it's because I had chosen a particular number because I was comparing myself to someone else or wanted to prove myself in some way. In short, my financial goals were often externally motivated. I was listening to my inner good girl who wanted to keep up and look good and had totally lost track of how I wanted to feel.

When I start with the feeling and base my goal around that (whether it's to do with my business, health or relationships), I find that I reach my aim much more easily. This is because I'm tuning into my unbound self – the part of me that doesn't care about how I look to others; she simply cares about being true to me and feeling the best that I can in each moment.

When I work with clients we look at ways they can begin to access their unbound-self-goal-feeling right away, helping them to bypass the inner good girl.

Want to lose weight so you can feel more confident? Let's turn that on its head and look at how you can feel more confident right now. Maybe you have a particular outfit that makes you feel fabulous, so you can get that out of your wardrobe and tap into your confidence that way? How about trying out a new class or activity to take a step out of your comfort zone? It may feel scary at first, but I guarantee this will grow your sense of confidence.

Want to make more money so you can feel free? How can you begin to build a sense of freedom right away? Maybe you can change up your routine, so you have time each day to do something you love to do (even if it's just for 30 minutes)? Perhaps you can book a weekend away, take yourself to a coffee shop to work on a creative project for the afternoon, or schedule a luxurious spa day?

Your inner good girl will tell you that 'good things come to those who wait' and make you believe that you have to work really hard to reach your goals. But your unbound self knows that there will always be something you can do to access the feeling that underlies your goal straight away.

So, how do you know whether you've been setting good girl goals? Here's a simple exercise to help you.

Exercise – A fail-safe way to check if you've set a good girl goal

1. Pick a specific goal that you're working towards at the moment.

2. Say the goal to yourself, either out loud or silently in your mind, and

notice how you feel in your body. What physical sensations do you feel as you focus on your goal?

3. Do these physical sensations feel expansive or constricting?

You will probably be able to tell this straight away, as I'm pretty sure you're tuned into what feels great and what feels blah. If you're not sure, focus on something you know you feel good about and notice how that feels in your body, then focus on something you feel icky about and notice how that feels. You can then compare these sensations to those you experience when you think about your goal.

For me, when I think about an unbound self goal, I get an expansive tug forward from my belly. When I focus on a good girl goal, I get a constricted feeling in my belly, like it's shrinking in on itself. (You can tell that my belly is my emotional compass, can't you?)

If you find that you've set yourself a good girl goal, you can decide whether you want to shift it so it feels more unbound, OR let it go completely. (Remember, the way to tune into an unbound self goal is to think about how you want to feel.)

Whether you decide to let the goal go completely, or shift it into a more unbound goal, you're back in the driving seat!

Btw it's fine to feel scared when you're thinking about a particular goal. Fear is completely normal when you're moving out of your comfort zone. Again you can check in with your body to see whether it's an expansive, scary-but-good kinda fear or a constrictive, I'm-only-doing-this-because-I-feel-I-should fear.

'Ultimately we know deeply that the other side of every fear is freedom.'
Marilyn Ferguson

Moving away from good girl goals and towards unbound self goals is key to creating the life and business you truly desire and as you move through this book, you'll find it easier and easier to tune into what you really want.

Appreciating how far you've come and celebrating your successes

Another good girl quality is not taking the time to appreciate and acknowledge your successes when you do achieve a goal.

When I surveyed my community, 26% said that when they achieve a goal, they immediately turn their attention to what's next rather than enjoying the moment.

Here are some of the examples given:

When I wrote my first books, as soon as they were published I went onto the next one instead of really cherishing the fact that they were out in the big wide world. Big mistake!

Completed BA degree and was ready to sign up next day for my masters!!

I get this completely! I've been a life-long achievement junkie. I was always working towards one goal or another and as soon as I achieved it, I would immediately think, 'What's next?'

When I think back over the goals I've achieved in the past (whether personal or professional), I've very rarely taken a moment to appreciate what I've done. When I got my degree, I was immediately thinking about the job I wanted.

When I qualified as a financial adviser, I immediately set myself a new goal of working towards a specialised investment qualification. When I retrained as a hypnotherapist, I worked my way through one therapy qualification after another – counselling, coaching, Neuro Linguistic Programming, Emotional Freedom Technique – and then as I built my practice, I moved from one business training to another.

Even when I got married in 2012, I didn't take time to appreciate this major life event; I was straight back to work and into the process of buying a house.

The inner good girl's eyes are always firmly on the road ahead. She's always thinking about the next goal, the next achievement, the next step on the imaginary ladder. She's always aiming higher and away from where she is right now.

But why? Why do so many of us suffer from this need to keep moving from one goal to another? It all comes down to a lack of self-belief. Somewhere along the line the inner good girl has received the message that she's not good enough and this has led her to question her self-worth.

When you did the exercise to discover where your inner good girl came from, it's likely that the key experience involved feeling not good enough in some way. This limiting belief is so incredibly common amongst women and its impact is huge. I've seen it time and time again, both in myself and my clients. For many of us, it gets to the point where we're thinking, 'Surely it can't be this old "I'm not good enough" belief coming up again?'

But it does. And the inner good girl is particularly sensitive to 'I'm not good enough'. If she gets the slightest sense that someone is questioning her enough-ness, she either retreats completely or goes into overdrive, trying to prove them wrong.

This is where the constant need to achieve comes in. Because she never quite feels good enough, the inner good girl is constantly on the move, jumping without a break from one goal to the next. And of course, this is exhausting.

One of the keys to happiness is to appreciate where you are right now, the successes you've already created in your life. But the inner good girl never gets to experience this as her eyes are firmly fixed on the next prize (whatever that may be). This leaves you with a constant feeling of dissatisfaction and striving.

If you want to feel good about yourself, you need to create a practice of regular reflection to appreciate how far you've come. It's great to have goals as a focus for what you want to move towards, but they're meaningless if you don't create a space to acknowledge and celebrate your successes.

Exercise – Acknowledging and celebrating your successes

Take out your journal and give yourself at least 30 minutes to do this exercise.

Think back over the past twelve months and write down everything you've achieved during this time. Your first thought might be 'Well, there's nothing', but I guarantee that's not true and that's why I want you to spend at least 30 minutes on this.

Think about the different areas of your life – work, family, relationships, social, health, financial, spiritual – and ask yourself these questions:

What new things have I tried?

What's gone well in each of these areas?

What's made me feel good?

What have I received positive feedback for?

Where have I made a difference?

What's felt like a win?

Start writing. Big or small, everything counts. Once you start, more and more successes will come to you (believe me!). If you find you're struggling with this, enlist a friend to help you. Very often someone who's close to you will be able to see your achievements more clearly than you can.

Once you have your list, look back over it and notice how you feel. Say to yourself, 'I'm proud of everything I've achieved over the past year. I'm choosing to acknowledge and appreciate my successes from now on.'

Choose a way to celebrate your achievements. You could go out for dinner, book a weekend away, go to the spa – whatever you would like to do. If your inner good girl tries to chime in and tell you not to bother, let her know (politely) that you're choosing to celebrate how far you've come. She can either join you or stay at home in protest, but you're celebrating regardless of what she chooses to do. (I bet she wants to come with you! This is great learning for her.)

After this initial success appreciation, I invite you to make it a regular practice. Each week, put aside a time to acknowledge and celebrate your wins and what's gone well. I tend to do this on a Friday afternoon and have a weekly appreciation/celebration thread over in my Facebook Group, Unbound Living (so please feel free to join me over there! The link to join is: www.facebook.com/groups/unboundwithnicolahumber). But you can do this whenever feels good for you. Just make sure you do it! This is non-negotiable (and fortunately, it's fun!).

STEP SIX – PEOPLE-PLEASING – WHEN YOU CAN'T SAY 'NO'

Oh, this is a classic, isn't it?

I've worked with countless clients over the years who felt unable to say 'No' to requests for their time and energy, from their families, friends and colleagues.

I've seen it in workplaces. 'Can you just help me with this?' (And four hours later you're still plugging away at this task you were assured would only take a few minutes of your time.)

Socially. 'Do you want to come to my party?' (And although you would rather stick pins in your eyes, you agree to go and dread it for weeks beforehand.)

Romantically. 'Can I take you on another date?' (And you say yes, even though you feel like you've just lost three hours of your life that you will never get back and know that he's 100% not your ideal man.)

The inability to say 'No' shows up everywhere. Because your inner good girl hates to say 'No'. She's been told it's rude. She's been told it's selfish to put her own needs before others, so she's a 'Yes' girl all the way.

When I asked my community whether they have trouble saying 'No' to others (even when they know they really don't want to do something), 47% said this was something they often struggled with.

Here are some of the specific examples they gave:

Right now it's about watching a film on TV which I know isn't right for me – usually violent or crime or horror – and after much pleading I give in to 'please' and hate it. Then I get cross with myself for not sticking with my inner knowing.

I'm doing work for a client that is poorly paid, but I've been with them a long time. The original people I liked and have loyalty to have left and therefore I don't have the same feeling of being valued. I want to tell them that I don't want to work for them any more, but I find I keep putting it off because it seems rude or ungrateful.

Simple things, like when I'm in the middle of a task and my partner can't find something that isn't urgent, but instead of saying to him that I'll look for it later when I have time, I stop what I'm doing to help him.

I'm often asked for vouchers for raffle prizes in my business. Although it doesn't cost anything to do and they aren't redeemed very often, it's just a hassle. They don't lead to future business so I'd just like to stop.

I do this with work. I make a decision to cut my hours and then I book somebody in. I then regret it and don't give the person my all and then I feel bad. It's a vicious cycle!

A substantial 58% of respondents said they often like to please others. And to tell you the truth I thought this was one area where I had it nailed. I've generally been pretty good at saying 'No' if I didn't want to do something. Maybe not always, but most of the time.

I would tell my clients that being selfish wasn't necessarily a bad thing. When we look after ourselves and make sure that our own needs are met, we have more energy for others in our lives. I had this spiel off pat. 1–0 to me against my inner good girl!

But recently I had an inner revelation (which was one of the inspirations for me to write this book actually). I realised that although I was good at saying 'No' to other people and keeping clear boundaries, I was terrible at saying 'No' to my inner good girl.

As soon as she got an idea to do something, I would be jumping in like a shot.

'Hey Nicola, you should write a blog post about this.' Yeah, you're so right. I'm on it.

'Nicola, you need to launch an online program. Everyone else is doing it. Hurry up!' Oh yes. I definitely should. I'll start creating the sales page right away.

'Nicola, you really need a clear fitness goal. How about signing up for that half-marathon?' Oh yes, I really should. I'll start my training plan now.

My inner good girl would say 'Jump' and I was leaping immediately.

And I've only recently realised this – I just haven't been able to say 'No' to my inner good girl.

You see, I assumed that all of these ideas were inspiration and I had to do them as soon as they came to me, even if it meant it was too much for me.

So I did. And I often ended up feeling completely overwhelmed and burned out. Because that's what happens when we don't say 'No' enough. We get tired, depleted, broken down. And then we're no good to anyone.

The lesson I've learned over the past six months is that it's okay to take a pause when I get an idea to do something. I can take some time, let the notion breathe and check in to get a feel of whether it's coming from my inner good girl or my unbound self.

And I can tell you, this has been a game-changer for me.

As a fellow creative (and btw, we're all creative, okay? More on that later in the book), I'm sure you get lots of ideas all the time. And I see so many women jumping from one thing to the next, always looking ahead and never taking the time to really finish what they started, meaning they constantly feel like failures. And, yep, that was me too.

But do you know what? You don't have to do everything all at once. You don't have to do everything that's asked of you. You don't have to do anything at all if you don't want to. And that in itself is a biggie. The inner good girl often has a huge issue with being seen as 'lazy'.

Relax. Put your feet up. Read a book. Go for a walk. (And turn the volume down on your inner good girl if she berates you for this.)

Hint: One of my best antidotes for inner-good-girl-itis is to read anything by SARK. She's a complete genius and a huge advocate of taking a nap. One of her mottos is to 'Practice extravagant lounging'. She's SO unbound. Go read Succulent Wild Woman by SARK if you haven't already (after you've read this, of course!). Check out my recommended reading list at the end of this book.

You'll know if you're a yes girl as you're reading this. And it will be showing up in some way in your life – through exhaustion, irritation, depression, weight gain or some other manifestation.

I once worked with a hypnotherapy client who came to me for help with weight loss. It was clear that she was an emotional eater and also that she was the one in her family who would always say 'Yes' to others' demands.

At first, she couldn't imagine beginning to say 'No'. I encouraged her to experiment with it and the change was remarkable.

Instead of being the one who always helped her elderly parents as well as helping her sister with her business, she started to say 'No' occasionally. She spent more time reading (which she loved and hadn't done for years). She put her feet up more often (which had been unheard of in the past) and the weight dropped off, really naturally, with no effort on her part (apart from saying 'No'). She stopped listening to her inner good girl and it was as if a weight was lifted from her shoulders (and her belly).

In his book, *When the Body Says No*, Gabor Mate M.D. says that 'When we have been prevented from learning how to say no, our bodies may end up saying it for us.' He gives many examples and case-studies of illnesses and medical conditions that have been brought on by chronic people-pleasing. Check out the recommended reading list at the end of this book for more details.

'When one is pretending, the entire body revolts.'
Anais Nin

When you consistently and persistently put others' needs above your own, you deny yourself and it will show up either physically, emotionally or psychologically.

The fact is, you are not meant to be constantly giving in to others' needs and wants. You are here to be yourself. It really is that simple. But the inner good girl seems to have forgotten this.

What beliefs have to do with it

So, why is people-pleasing such a big issue for many of us?

Very often it's because there is some kind of script running that's leading us to believe that fitting in, being 'nice' and pleasing others is more important than our own needs. Your beliefs are the lens through which you see the world. They shape your perception. And the inner good girl has very often picked up beliefs that limit and constrict in some way.

Many of the beliefs that we carry through our lives were formed when we were very young. These key experiences, like the one that came to mind when you looked at when your inner good girl was formed, prompt us to make decisions about ourselves and our place in the world. These decisions take the form of beliefs that then impact on the way we interact with others.

Common beliefs that lead to people-pleasing are those such as:

'I'm unloveable' – therefore, I have to do everything I can to please others and make them like me.

'I'm not good enough' – so I have to go the extra mile to prove myself.

'I'm not worthy' – so I have to say 'Yes' to every request to show I can be of value.

Sometimes these underlying scripts or beliefs can be a little more subtle though. I recently discovered a surprising limiting belief that had been shaping my interactions with others.

As I had been connecting with my own inner good girl and working through my own healing process, I tuned into a memory from when I was about four years old. I had forgotten this particular experience and the details weren't overly clear, but I remembered being a little girl at my grandmother's house in the New Forest and I had just been shouted at by my dad.

I couldn't remember exactly what had happened, but I knew it was something to do with me being told off for being noisy. The memory that came to mind was little Nicola on her own, by my grandmother's fire, feeling upset and confused because Dad had just shouted at her and she couldn't understand why.

As I worked with the memory and connected with little Nicola, I realised that in that moment she had made a decision that 'I make people angry'. Dad's response just didn't make sense to her, so she figured that just the act of being herself made people angry.

As I reflected on this, I realised that this belief very much tied in with the classroom experience where my inner good girl was fixed in place. In that experience, I had thought that I had made the teacher angry, so it reinforced this underlying belief.

'I make people angry.'

Suddenly the way I saw my place in the world and the way I interacted with others made a lot more sense to me.

One of my tendencies has been to constantly monitor what I say to others. Whether it was someone close to me, a new acquaintance or someone serving me coffee, I carefully chose my words before speaking to make sure that what I was saying was 'acceptable'. I would often hold back from speaking at all. And this constant self-monitoring had been exhausting and confusing to me.

In my business it showed up in the way I communicated with clients and my online community. I would hold back from sending emails or posting on social media because unconsciously I was worried that I would 'make people angry'. I somehow disregarded the fact that what I had to share and the work I do is hugely beneficial to others and held back from communicating.

This fear that I might make people angry meant that I was overly conscious of pleasing others. Over the years I shaped and moulded myself to be as inoffensive as possible. I would say 'Yes' to others to keep the peace and generally be a nice girl. And by being overly aware of the possibility that I could make people angry, I held on to a lot of anger myself (more on that in Step Eleven).

This kind of self-monitoring (which runs alongside people-pleasing) is very common in the inner good girl. And it can demand a huge amount of energy.

So, what are the beliefs that have been shaping your world? What are the stories you've been telling yourself that have been limiting your perception and increasing your desire to please others?

The easiest way to discover them is to ask your inner good girl.

Use the Meeting your inner good girl visualisation from Step Two and during that interaction, ask her how she feels about herself and her place in the world.

When we try to think of these limiting beliefs with the conscious mind, we can second-guess ourselves and think too logically, too much like an adult. The kind of beliefs that lead to people-pleasing were formed when we were children, so you need to connect with that very young part of you – the inner good girl.

Why is it important to bring these beliefs into your awareness?

Well, as you've seen throughout this chapter, these old scripts have a huge impact on the way we relate to others. Although these beliefs may have served a purpose when we were very young, they limit and restrict us as adults. Once you shine the light of awareness on these inner good girl beliefs, they naturally begin to dissolve.

Whenever I notice a tendency to hold back or monitor myself now, I recognise that this comes from a very young part of me and her fear that I might make someone angry. That knowledge allows me to stand firmly in my adult self and make an empowered choice about what to say or do.

Exercise – Permission to say 'No'

So, where in your life are you saying 'Yes' (either to yourself or others) when you really want to say 'No'?

For the next 24 hours, give yourself a break from saying 'Yes' to any requests, invitations, opportunities or impulses. You can simply say, 'That sounds interesting. I'll check my diary and get back to you.'

Notice how it feels to delay making a decision. It's possible that you may experience some resistance to this and that's okay. Know that it's your inner good girl wanting to jump in and please others.

Choose to see this as an experiment. I always find that by approaching new ideas or behaviours as an experiment, it's easier to try them out.

As any requests, opportunities or ideas come to you, simply make a note of them. By giving yourself permission to delay your decision-making, you're creating a space to tune into your unbound self and make a choice that truly serves you.

At the end of your 24 hours, take some time to look at your list of requests etc. Go through each one and check in with how you feel about it. (It can help to tune into your body for this, using the same technique I suggested in the 'Are you setting good girl goals?' exercise.)

Ask yourself these questions:

Do I want to do this?

Do I need to do this?

How would I feel if I chose to do this?

How would I feel if I chose not to do this?

Give yourself permission to make spacious, unbound decisions.

It's likely that you will decide to say 'No' to things that you initially wanted to say 'Yes' to. And that's okay.

Affirm to yourself, 'It's okay for me to say "No". I make choices that support me.'

Make this your new mantra and experiment with saying 'No' more often.

STEP SEVEN – MONEY STUFF AND BEING OPEN TO RECEIVE

Oh, this is a big one! Where to begin?

Until I started my business, I really didn't think a whole lot about money and my attitudes towards it (even though I worked in finance). I had enough to get by very comfortably and had received steady salary increases over the years.

But when I started my business, suddenly the way I received money changed and it was all down to me. I got to choose how much I was going to charge my clients and there was going to be a direct exchange of money. I had to place a value on my services and this brought up so many questions for me, especially when I was starting out as a new hypnotherapist.

'Can I do this?'

'Will someone actually pay for this?'

'How much should I charge?'

'What if that's too much?'

'What if someone asks for their money back?'

And the classic, 'Am I good enough?'

It all felt so personal. I knew that I had to create a sustainable income and that if I didn't value what I had to offer, then no-one else would. But my inner good girl had so many issues about money, which were now rising to the surface.

First and foremost, she felt it was wrong to talk about money openly. This meant that I would often resist talking about my fees and when a client asked me, 'How much will it cost?', I'd awkwardly state my hourly rate, then jump in with a discount before they had even had a chance to respond.

My inner good girl had picked up the belief that it was rude to talk about money when I was very young and this belief bubbled away in the background as I struggled over setting my prices and asking to be paid. And of course, this discomfort around talking about money is not unique to me.

In November 2015, Kate Winslet was being interviewed about the gender pay-gap and openly stated that she found the whole debate uncomfortable. She felt it was 'vulgar' to talk publicly about money. And she was simply echoing the beliefs of many women: 'It's vulgar to talk about money. Good girls keep their money stuff to themselves.'

Money mindset became one of my specialities after working through my own 'money stuff' and I've found that very often women are far happier to talk about sex than money. It's a taboo subject. But inequality thrives on secrecy. When we don't know what others are being paid, we have no idea whether we're receiving less. And because money is often seen as taboo, we tend to keep quiet about it. We keep our money stuff to ourselves and that can lead to stress, anxiety and fear. So many women take a back seat when it comes to money and let someone else handle it (usually a man), because they're scared of money and being open about it.

Again, secrecy breeds fear.

And this was all a huge learning curve for me when I started my own business. My inner good girl wanted me to play it safe, to charge the going rate, the average, so I did and this felt nice and comfortable. 'Playing it safe' is a typical inner good girl tactic. She doesn't like to put her head above the parapet or be seen to 'make a fuss' (as she would put it).

This is in contrast to a male hypnotherapist I met on a training course a couple of years ago. He told me that when he started out he immediately began to charge more than any other hypnotherapists in his area (about £50 an hour more than his hypnotherapy tutor!). I was awe-struck.

He quite simply knew that if he valued his services highly, then his potential clients would too. And that proved to be the case, as he now has a thriving Harley Street practice and regularly works with A-list clients. There was certainly no inner good girl holding him back!

Underneath this discomfort around talking about and asking for money lies the limiting belief that money is 'bad' in some way. The inner good girl often picks up this belief as she's growing up – from her parents, grandparents, teachers, the church and society in general.

Many of us receive negative messages about money when we're young and the inner good girl is particularly sensitive to these. Being the good girl that she is, she certainly does not want to be associated with anything other people see as 'bad' in any way.

And when I say we receive negative messages, I don't mean that anyone actually said to you 'Money is bad' in so many words (however, it's not beyond the realms of possibility that someone might have said this to you). You're likely to have picked up a belief that money is bad in subtler ways.

Maybe you often saw your parents arguing about money when you were growing up and picked up the idea that money was a source of conflict and stress?

Perhaps your family criticised rich people, suggesting that they were arrogant, that they only got their wealth by treading on others or that they were just plain evil?

Maybe you saw how your parents struggled to make money and they told you that it's really hard work to make enough to live on?

There are many ways to receive the idea that money is bad in some way. And the media often backs this up with stories about 'greedy fat cats' and wealthy people wasting money on extravagant lifestyles whilst the 'rest of us' struggle to get by.

And of course, money isn't inherently good or bad. Money just is. But we often find it hard to see money in this neutral way. And the inner good girl struggles with this very much.

On one hand, she wants to be seen to do well, to achieve and to be successful. But on the other hand, she doesn't want to be seen as a money-grabbing bitch (and that's exactly how she imagines people will perceive her if she has 'too much'). How much is 'too much'? Well, of course, the inner good girl has no idea. But in order to make sure she doesn't break through the 'too much' level, she tends to hold herself back and often self-sabotage will come into play.

I've seen this throughout my life. At times when I've started to do well financially, I've often found myself sabotaging that success – entering destructive relationships, getting sick, backing off from opportunities. In his book, *The Big Leap*, Gay Hendricks calls this self-sabotage an Upper Limit Problem. And it doesn't just happen financially. Ever had a huge argument with your partner when things had been going really well? That could well be an Upper Limit Problem too.

Hint: If you haven't read The Big Leap, *search it out. It's packed full of insights and I recommend it to many of my clients. Check out my recommended reading list at the end of this book for more details.*

The inner good girl tends to be in this constant cycle of doing well followed by some form of self-sabotage. And she often holds herself back from opportunities that could lead to making more money because she has an underlying belief that 'money is bad'.

I wonder if you've seen this in yourself?

Exercise – Your money beliefs

So, what are your beliefs around money? Let's bring some of those inner good girl money beliefs into your awareness. (Because, remember, awareness is always the first step to change.)

To do this, get your notebook out and on a new page, complete the following statements:

Money is ......

To be wealthy, I would have to ....

If I was rich, ...

I was always told that to make money ....

I feel .... talking about money.

Rich people are ....

Don't think too much about what to write, just go with whatever comes to mind.

As you read back through what you've written, notice whether the words you've chosen feel expansive or constricting. The statements you've come up with are clues to your underlying beliefs about money and wealth. So, are these beliefs likely to support your ability to create wealth or restrict it?

Now, I'm not saying that everyone wants to be super-rich (or should want to be), but when we have limiting beliefs running around money, these can impact on more than your bank balance. Negative money beliefs can stop you from reaching your full potential and being your brightest, most brilliant self.

So, once you've brought these inner good girl money beliefs into your awareness, you can begin to shift them. There are two steps to this.

1. Look for evidence that your limiting money belief is not true.

As the wonderful human beings that we are, we tend to only notice the evidence that supports what we already believe to be true.

So, if you have a belief that money is bad in some way, you will naturally notice all of the evidence that backs this up – stories in the newspaper about greedy bankers and lottery winners who go off the rails.

But there will also be plenty of evidence to challenge your old beliefs. Stories about people who give money to good causes and past experiences where you've used money to do something wonderful for yourself or others.

There will *always* be evidence to support both sides of the coin and it's completely your choice which you choose to focus on.

So, take one belief at a time and consciously look for evidence that challenges it. Write this down and notice how you feel as you begin to change your focus.

2. Create your unbound money beliefs.

Once you've begun to challenge your inner good girl money beliefs, you can begin to write a new money story for yourself.

With each of your old money beliefs, think about how you could choose to rewrite it in a more positive, expansive way.

For example, if your old belief was 'Money is bad', your new, unbound belief might be:

Money empowers me to give to myself and others freely.

Or,

Money is a tool for good.

Or,

Money helps me to be my fullest self.

The important thing is to choose words that feel good for you, words that make you feel more connected to your unbound self.

3. When you have your new, positive beliefs, you can begin to use them as affirmations and mantras. This will help to embed these new ideas in your powerful subconscious mind.

An affirmation or mantra is simply a positive statement that you repeat regularly, either out loud or silently in your mind.

You can incorporate your chosen affirmations and mantras into your daily life in a number of different ways:

- Say them to yourself (either out loud or in your mind) just before you get up in the morning and last thing at night before you go to sleep. Your subconscious mind is particularly open at these times.
- Write them down and place them somewhere you will see them often throughout the day.
- Create a screensaver for your phone, tablet or laptop with your chosen affirmation or mantra.
- Say them to yourself as you brush your teeth.
- Say them out loud as you are driving or stuck in traffic
- Say them in your mind as you're standing in a queue.
- Say them to yourself as you're working out or walking. Combining affirmations with physical movement is particularly powerful.

You may find that these new statements don't feel completely true to you initially. That's completely natural – creating new beliefs can take time and repetition. Keep going and, combined with the other work you're doing in this book, your new beliefs will start to become reality for you.

Are you open to receive?

The inner good girl operates on the basis that you should have as little impact on others as possible. You should be able to do everything for yourself and asking for help is a sign of weakness.

She believes that you shouldn't have to ask for anything. One of her key drivers is not to put anyone out (or not to 'make a fuss' as she sees it).

This means she has a distinct lack of receive-ability.

When I asked the question, 'What does the term "good girl" mean to you?' on my Facebook page, Clare wrote:

For me, it's feeling uncomfortable/troublesome asking for or receiving help; a 'good girl' doesn't bother anybody! For instance, feeling dehydrated today at a client site and without access to refreshments, I found myself getting nauseous and headachey because I didn't want to interrupt the session/put anyone out to track down a glass of water.

Similarly, a family member I was visiting recently offered to pick me up from the airport: I felt awkward and guilty for the whole car journey instead of feeling grateful I didn't have to take public transport and got to spend extra time with them. So daft when I think about it!

And that's the thing – when we look back at situations like this we *do* feel daft, but I'm sure we've all had times when we've been in groups and not wanted to ask for some water or pop to the toilet, because we didn't want to put anyone out. I know I have. Many, many times.

This ties in with not being able to say 'No'. The inner good girl is always thinking about the other person she's in relation to and how to meet their needs, all the time undermining her own. It's classic people-pleasing behaviour. And whenever we deny our own needs, we're sending a message to ourselves that we're not worthy.

Here are some other typical examples of not being open to receive (all of which I've experienced myself):

A friend offers to pay for coffee or lunch, but your inner good girl is adamant that you need to pay your share. In fact, she would prefer that you pay for the whole bill because it's rude to accept random gifts from others. The inner good girl has to pay her way (or more than her way!).

In business, the inner good girl will discount her prices to make them more 'acceptable'. She doesn't want to stand out by asking for more, so she will put up with receiving less than she really wants (or less than she's worth), even when this means she can't live her life in the way she truly desires.

The inner good girl will not ask for help or support, even when she really needs it. She will say, 'No, I'm fine' (often through gritted teeth) and struggle on believing that she has to do everything herself. In fact, she believes it's selfish to look after herself and make her needs a priority.

The inner good girl has firmly closed the door on receiving. In fact, she equates 'receiving' of any kind as 'making a fuss'.

So if someone asks her what she would like to do, or where she would like to go, her stock response is, 'I don't mind. You choose.' Much easier to pass the decision back to someone else. God forbid the inner good girl should actually receive what she wants!

I've had countless 'good girls' come to see me as clients saying that they feel 'self-indulgent' for seeking help with issues that are limiting the way they live. In my work with them we have to deal with the guilt of asking for support before we even begin to look at the issue in hand.

When I started my business I had a strong belief that I had to do everything myself. As well as seeing clients, I was designing my website, marketing, doing the accounts and administration, copy-writing – everything that goes with running a small business. I thought I should be able to do it all myself and if I couldn't, there was something wrong with me.

I see this time and time again with other women business-owners. They wear themselves out, trying to do it all. It's the same with good girl mothers who feel it's a sign of failure to ask for help, like getting a cleaner or a child-minder. The inner good girl runs you ragged and every opportunity to receive is met with a firm, 'No thank you'.

In contrast the unbound self recognises that if someone offers your something, they actually want you to say, 'Yes'. The unbound self recognises the pleasure we all take in giving and having our gifts (whether it's time, money, support or listening) met with gratitude and appreciation. The unbound self knows there's no shame in saying, 'Actually, I'm struggling at the moment. Can you help me?' The unbound self is open to receive and because of that she's able to go through life feeling beautifully supported (and, as a consequence, more able to support others).

So, if you're feeling unsupported at the moment, ask yourself, 'Where am I closed off to receive?' Where are you battling on where you could really do with some help? Where are you putting the needs of others in front of your own?

Because if your inner good girl is keeping you closed off to receiving, you'll be feeling pretty darn resentful deep down.

And that's the thing. Your inner good girl wants you to be nice and helpful and polite, but deep down she's likely to be seething. She's tried to live her whole life based on sticking to the rules (more on this in the next chapter), being careful about how she's received, and it's left her exhausted and frustrated.

Exercise: Boost your receive-ability

For the next 24 hours, set your antennae and be on the lookout for any situation where you're closed off to receiving.

Commit to opening up to receive. Build your receiving muscle!

Here are some examples that may help you:

Accept any offers of help and support.

Ask for what you need – the glass of water, a hand cooking dinner, an introduction to someone who can help you with a particular project. Affirm to yourself, 'It's okay to ask for what I need.'

Graciously accept compliments and positive feedback. Notice any temptation to say, 'Oh, it was nothing' or 'This old thing?' All you have to say is 'Thank you'. No deflecting!

Say 'Yes' when a friend offers to pay for coffee/lunch/dinner.

Make clear offers to potential clients or collaborators and then be quiet. Notice any impulse to jump in with a discount or justification. Bite your tongue (gently, of course!), sit on your hands and simply wait for their response.

If someone asks you what you want to do or where you want to go, make a decision. Even if you feel like you've got no real preference, choose!

Again, this may well feel uncomfortable. You're beginning to change habits that have likely been ingrained since childhood. Small steps my friend, small steps towards your glorious open-to-receive unbound self!

STEP EIGHT – CREATIVITY AND PERFECTIONISM

In this step we're looking at creativity and how the inner good girl shows up in this area. This is one aspect of our lives that can often be neglected. When we're children, being creative tends to be a big part of our lives. When we're young, we draw, paint, write, make and imagine as a matter of course. We don't stop to question, 'Is this good enough?' or 'Am I creative?' We simply get on and enjoy playing and creating for the fun of it.

But as we get older, doubts start to kick in. Maybe Mum doesn't respond as positively as you had expected to a painting you bring home from school? Or a teacher criticises your efforts in an art class? Or you don't get picked for a role in the school play? And with each experience like this, your inner good girl starts to shut off from her creative world.

She tells herself that painting is silly or just for kids. She turns her attention to other, 'more important' things, tasks where she can receive the recognition she craves. The inner good girl has no time or inclination to do things she believes she can't do well. Unless she's formally acknowledged as a 'creative person' through qualifications or her career, then any form of creativity is likely to play a back seat (or no role at all) in her life.

I get this.

As I was growing up and for much of my life I never thought of myself as creative. As soon as my inner good girl took hold at school, I tended to concentrate on subjects I knew I could do well at – maths, English, science, languages. All of the more academic subjects were okay. They were safe. Anything vaguely artistic felt too risky.

Although I loved writing stories when I was little (more on this later in the chapter), any writing I did after the age of about ten was purely non-fiction. (And actually that carries on until today. I'd love to write fiction. It's a dream of mine. But I struggle to know where to start.)

I enjoyed being in school plays at infants and junior school, but couldn't imagine performing in any way again until I got well into my thirties. Up until that point, my inner good girl was taking herself way too seriously.

A Greek odyssey

Actually it was on a self-development holiday in Greece that I began to tap back into my creativity. It was a holiday I had dreamed of taking for years: a week on a Greek island at a holistic centre and the chance to pick two or three different courses to try out new activities.

I had finally plucked up courage to go, after years of looking at the brochure and website. As I arrived on the island, I told myself I would probably stick to courses I felt 'safe' with – maybe windsurfing or yoga. But as we were on the coach driving to the centre where we would be staying, the guide encouraged us to take courses we would never usually imagine trying, activities that maybe scared us.

In that moment something in my unbound self stirred.

As I sat in the welcome talk that evening, listening to the different facilitators describing the courses they offered, I chose to stay open to the possibilities. And rather than sticking with the 'safe' options I had imagined I would take, I decided to go with the guided writing course I was intrigued by and a drawing course.

As I look back, I can see this was a turning point for me. This one-week holiday moved me onto a different path in life. The guided writing course I had been called to was my first experience of both inner child work and connecting with my higher self. And I loved the drawing course. I realised that I could actually create a drawing that pleased me and, more importantly, I enjoyed the process.

Also during that week, I had my first experience of performing since school. I knew that there was going to be a cabaret at the end of the week where anyone could get up and do their bit. I had seen the details on the company's website and before I'd even left home, I had completely ruled out taking part in the show. My inner good girl had kicked in and made the idea of it seem ridiculous. But when I arrived at the centre, one of the women I got to know suggested that a group of us put a song and dance act together. I was terrified at the thought of it, but agreed.

So at the end of the week we found ourselves doing a chaotic performance of 'Get Happy' complete with brooms in our hands (as my group was collectively responsible for sweeping the centre each day). And I loved it! I felt so exhilarated to be on stage, performing in front of a group of accepting, supportive people.

Hint: A feeling of exhilaration is a clear sign that you're connecting with your unbound self.

Again, this was a breakthrough for me. Since then, I've been far happier to take part in performances of all kinds, whether that's public speaking or being part of a group Burlesque show. (FYI, my Burlesque name is Gracie Galore.) My inner good girl has learned over time that it's okay to do things just for the fun of it. And it's even okay to make a fool of myself.

And that's the thing. The reason why many of us lose touch with our creativity is that we worry about 'getting it right'. The inner good girl tends to be a perfectionist and it's pretty hard (if not impossible) to get creativity perfect.

You might be reading this and thinking, 'Well, I'm not creative anyway. I might as well just skip this step and move on to the next one.' And if you are, know that it's your inner good girl kicking in. As a human being (and I'm assuming that you're human?), you can't help but be creative.

The definition of creative is:

> *Relating to or involving the use of the imagination or original ideas to create something.*

And there are two things I can absolutely guarantee:

1. You use your imagination on a daily basis.
2. You are constantly creating something.

Now maybe you're shaking your head and thinking, 'Nope! Not me.'

Well, I beg to differ, my friend. Your imagination is constantly being used as you live your life. Before you do anything, you have to imagine it first. When you're thinking about what to have for dinner, where to go on holiday, which route to take to work – all of this happens in your imagination first.

So your life is an act of constant creation. Each decision you make, each time you try something different, every preference you state – it's ALL creative.

So, you may not identify with the idea of being creative, but you inherently are. It's very possible however that your inner good girl has stifled your creativity. Maybe she's narrowed the range of original ideas you're willing to try out?

Perhaps she's kept you on the 'safe' path? It's okay. Because as you begin to recognise and acknowledge your creativity, your inner good girl will become more fluid around this.

The very process you're working through right now as you read this book is creative. I'm asking you to imagine interactions with your inner good girl and unbound self, write imaginary letters, make believe that you're taking your inner good girl for a walk. It's possible that you haven't used your creative imagination in this way since you were a child. So, how does it feel?

When I'm using these kind of techniques with clients, particularly in hypnotherapy, they'll often express a fear that they're just 'making it up'. Well of course they're making it up, if by 'making it up' they mean harnessing the power of their imaginations. When you tap into your imagination, you're tapping into your subconscious. It all comes from within you and it all comes for a reason.

This process of 'making it up' is what allows healing to occur.

Healing is creative.

Creativity is healing.

Exercise – How are you already using your creativity?

Your first exercise this week is to notice all the ways you're being creative in your life already.

What you focus on flourishes. So the more you acknowledge any ways you express your creativity right now, the more creative you will become. And more importantly, the more creative you will feel.

Your inner good girl will begin to get used to the idea that you are creative and you will feel more connected with your unbound self. It's a win–win.

So take some time now. Sit down with your journal and begin to focus on all the ways you are creative already.

As you sit in front of a blank page, you may very well experience resistance to this.

Your inner good girl may kick in with the idea that you're simply not creative, so why bother with this exercise?

It's okay.

Just put pen to paper and begin.

To help you, here's what comes to mind for me.

How do I express my creativity already?

- The way I work with my clients.
- The way I've purposefully chosen to create my life and business.
- The clothes I choose to wear each day – the scarf I'm wearing right now as I write this.
- The inspirational meme I've just created to post on Facebook.
- The regular blogs I write.
- The content I create for my online community.
- Whenever I choose to dance in the kitchen or bathroom.
- The photos I often snap as I'm out walking.
- The different routes I take on my daily walk.
- The stories I create in my head about other people I see and about my own future.
- The way I prefer to cook without a recipe.

- Whenever I decide to take a different class or activity.
- When I imagine that the droplets of water hanging from the tree branches outside are like jewels.
- The words I choose to use when I write or speak.

All of this is creative. And I must admit I found it hard to get going with this list (for many of the ideas my inner good girl chimed in and said, 'Well that's just stupid!'). But I kept going. And it feels good to acknowledge my creativity.

So, have a go. Spend at least fifteen minutes writing down a list of all the ways you are creative.

Notice how you feel as you do this.

Creativity and intuition

The truth is (and believe me, this is true), you probably generate hundreds of creative ideas daily. Creativity is closely linked to your intuition and your intuition is constantly guiding you.

But very often we don't listen. We don't listen to that knowing, wise and playful voice within us.

An idea springs to mind and the inner good girl constantly closes it down because she believes it's silly or risky or a thing someone else should be doing or something you're not qualified to do.

And the idea is lost.

As I'm writing this book, I'm re-reading Elizabeth Gilbert's *Big Magic* which is all about creativity and the mysteries of the creative process. In it she talks about inspiration and how it will come to you with an idea. If you respond positively, inspiration will work with you and bring more ideas. But if you close the door on the idea, inspiration will go elsewhere. It will turn to another, more willing, more receptive being.

So creativity is something to be nurtured, not feared. When you notice an idea pop into your head, feel grateful. Rather than saying, 'I can't do that', ask yourself the more expansive question, 'Why not?' and 'I wonder how I could do that?'

Hint: Asking a question, rather than making a statement, is a great way to tap into your unbound self. When you ask a question, you open the door of possibility and your subconscious mind cannot help but go looking for an answer. It may not come immediately, but it will come.

Maybe that particular idea isn't quite right for you, but maybe it is? Give it some space. Allow it to breathe. And then make your decision from a place of powerful expansion, rather than constrictive thinking.

Grow your ability to listen to your intuition. Grow your sense of possibility. Grow your creativity. Creativity is a magical doorway to the unbound realms of YOU. It's a sure-fire way to connect with your unbound self. And yes, as you stretch your creative muscle, you might feel exposed, or silly, or vulnerable, or scared, or unskilled, or clumsy, or all of the above. Simply acknowledge how you're feeling and keep going.

You're doing great.

The Wise Owl

Once upon a time, I wrote a story.

I was six or seven at the time and it was a story about a wise owl making the discovery that his true nature was to sleep during the day and come out at night.

(Previously he had been staying awake during the day to help the other animals.)

As a little girl, I was super-proud of this story. I knew it was good. And my teacher, Mrs Baker, took it home and typed it up for me, making it into a book (this was in the days before word processing programs, so she used an old-fashioned manual typewriter).

I was delighted with my 'book' and joyfully drew some illustrations of the wise owl to decorate the pages.

At the time I dreamed of being a writer; that was what I wanted to be when I grew up. I always had my nose in a book, reading and imagining.

I knew I was good at writing. And 'The Wise Owl' was part of the proof of that. But somewhere along the way, I lost that belief, that inner knowing, that I was good at writing. In fact, I lost the belief that I was good at anything.

Along the way, I picked up doubts and criticisms (both from myself and others).

Along the way I stopped creating. I stopped creating and started questioning – questioning my ability, questioning the innate talent that we all have and questioning whether I was good enough. And as I've been writing about throughout this chapter, this is something that happens to many of us. Many of us lose that inner belief that we are good enough – clever enough, creative enough, loveable enough – just as we are.

When I was going through some old papers recently I found that story I had written when I was a little girl – 'The Wise Owl'. As I sat and read the words, tears came to my eyes as I realised how beautiful the words were, how completely genius the story my younger self had written was and also how over the years I had lost that unrockable sense of belief in myself and what I had to offer to the world.

It was as if my six-year-old self was saying, 'Nicola, look what you can do! You're creative, you're funny, you're wise, you're loveable and you always have been. It's time to start being you again.' And this book is part of that process.

The inner good girl decides that in order to be acceptable, she needs to be perfect. And, of course, perfectionism is lethal when it comes to creativity.

Perfectionism and allowing yourself to be a beginner

When I asked my community whether they saw themselves as perfectionists and liked to get things right, 42% said this was often the case and 26% said always.

Some of the examples given were:

I worry my work is not good enough and will go over and over everything until I feel it is perfect – even if this causes other problems such as a late night or not feeding my kids until they are complaining!!!

I like my house to be immaculate – clean and tidy and I can't focus if it isn't. I spend a lot of time each week cleaning and tidying. I spend a lot of time writing and re-reading my blog posts before pushing the publish button. This means I write less posts!

I love to research. So I will spend a lot of time learning about something before I will even try it for the first time. And I get so disappointed if I don't get something right the first time.

I hate getting things wrong and sometimes don't even start for fear of failing. I want to start a business but I'm scared it will fail and I will look foolish to have even thought that I could do such a thing. I know I have done well in the past but my inner good girl says to stay safe, we don't step outside our boundaries (I know they are self-imposed and I have broken out before but right now we stay safe and play small). Arrghh!!!'

This belief that we need to be perfect stops many of us from trying anything new. In order to be creative, you need to allow yourself to make mistakes and often you need to go back to being a beginner.

This can feel deeply uncomfortable for those of us who generally choose to do only what we're good at, what we're experienced in doing.

Recently, I attended a creative healing workshop with a wonderful therapist, Charlotte Holst Schmid, who is local to me. Charlotte is a gifted jewellery-maker and part of the workshop involved making your own necklace.

I had never attempted to make jewellery before, so I was thrown into the situation of being a complete beginner. The process was fiddly and delicate, using tools and materials I wasn't familiar with. I noticed that I quickly became frustrated that my necklace wasn't taking shape in the way I had envisioned. But rather than indulging that frustration, I chose to take a deep breath and give myself permission to be the beginner. I allowed myself to enjoy the process (just as a child would) and in the end, I was delighted with what I had created. (In fact, I wear my necklace all the time now and I'm always proud to tell others that I made it myself.)

So, now I'm inviting you to move into beginner-mode.

Exercise – Expanding your sense of creativity

In this chapter, as you're making it your focus to expand your sense of creativity, I've put together some simple exercises for you to have fun with. (Fun being the operative word here.) Pick one or try them all. Maybe if you start with one, you'll feel compelled to try some others?

Notice which you feel drawn to.

And notice which you feel resistant to.

1. Create an image that expresses how you feel right now. Use lines, shapes and colours and whatever medium you have access to – paints, crayon, pens, pencils, even a biro! Don't feel you have to be literal. Just doodle and play and see what emerges on the page.

2. Write a one-page story about yourself imagining that you have magical super-powers. What do you do? Where do you go? What changes?

3. Take yourself on a photographic journey. Go for a walk and take photos of anything that captures your interest as you go. When you return, make your favourite photos into a collage. (www.picmonkey.com is a great, free online tool for this.)

4. Create an image that expresses either your inner good girl or unbound self (or both). Again, don't feel you have to be literal. Choose whatever colours and mediums seem to represent these different aspects of you.

5. Take some stones, leaves, flowers and twigs and make a sculpture in your garden or outdoor space that represents your unbound self. Know that this can be as permanent or impermanent as you choose. The important thing is to enjoy the process. Whatever you create is bringing you closer to your unbound self.

A note on the power of *focus*

As I look back on what I wrote at the beginning of this exercise, I particularly notice how I've used the words 'make it your focus'.

Make it your focus.

Four deceptively simple words, but they imply the following:

A)   You always have a choice.
B)   You can use that choice to decide what to focus on.

The whole point of this chapter is to guide you to focus on your innate creativity. It's already there within you. We're just shining a big ole torchlight on it in this step of the process.

So, why is this important?

Well the inner good girl tends to deny choices. She feels much safer when you're doing what you've always done or following a well-trodden path. And of course, this is death to creativity.

On the other hand, your unbound self is always open to a range of possibilities. She is much more receptive to creativity. And in each moment, you get to choose which of these different parts of you to move towards. In each moment, you have a choice. Nothing is set in stone. You can change your mind in a flash.

You get to choose what you focus on. And to what you turn your attention. And this is what makes your life creative. Choice.

STEP NINE – STICKING TO THE RULES

This has been a huge one for me. Despite all of the personal development work I've done over the years, I still find it difficult to break the rules.

I'm not talking about breaking the law here. I feel like I have to stick to every little rule there is – well, kind of, because the inner good girl is more complex than that of course.

Let me give you an example.

My sister and I went to see Deepak Chopra speak in 2014. It was at a large venue in London and after lunch we noticed that there were a number of empty seats nearer the front than we were. My sister immediately suggested that we go and sit in the better seats. Her thinking was 'Why not? If someone comes to claim them we can just move back again.'

In contrast, my thinking (or my inner good girl's response) was, 'But they're not our seats. It will be so embarrassing if we get caught.' (See how I was thinking like a child who didn't want to get told off for doing something naughty?)

In the end we did move to the closer seats, but my sister could tell that I felt so uncomfortable that we moved back to our 'proper' seats after a few minutes.

It's a running joke in my family that I don't like to break the rules. My sister, dad and husband are all far more rebellious. The fact is, if someone tells me I have to do something a particular way, I tend to do it, because my inner good girl has made it very clear over the years – good girls don't break the rules.

When I surveyed my community, nearly 53% of respondents said they often or always like to stick to the rules.

And these women are certainly not alone. In her book, *Lean In*, the Chief Operating Officer of Facebook, Sheryl Sandberg, talks about a speech she gave a few years ago. Towards the end of the speech she said that she would only take two more questions. It was a mixed audience of men and women, and after she had answered the said two questions, the women in the audience all put their hands down. But several of the men kept their hands up and Sandberg took their questions.

It was only after the speech when a woman came up to give her feedback that she realised what had happened. All of the women had stuck to the 'rules'; they had put their hands down like good girls. But many of the men had ignored the same rule and in keeping their hands up, they got their questions answered. Through stretching that rule, the men got their needs met.

There seems to be a greater tendency amongst women to stick to the rules. Our inner good girls believe it's important to do things the 'right' way (even when it comes at a cost to us). And if the inner good girl does break the rules (because everyone does sometimes), she will make you feel guilt and shame. Being caught out for doing something 'wrong' is pretty much unbearable for the inner good girl.

But who sets these rules? Well, they can be imposed from many directions – societal, cultural, religious and family rules.

As I look back I realise I've broken some seemingly biggies in the past.

Choosing to remain in a relationship with a man who was in prison.

Walking out of a job without giving any notice.

Having an affair with a married man.

When I've broken the rules in these BIG ways, I've been left feeling a huge amount of shame and questioning who I actually am, because these decisions that I made did not fit in any way with my established identity as a 'good girl'.

Even though I made all of these choices with the best of intentions and I can look back and see clearly that I was doing the best that I could at the time, my inner good girl gave me a super-hard time during and long after these life events.

Because only one thing really counts for the inner good girl – am I presenting myself as I should? Will what I'm doing or saying be deemed as 'acceptable' to others? She has an external focus, rather than tuning in to her inner compass.

The inner good girl plays by the rules and the rules she plays by aren't always obvious. Many of them are self-imposed and can include rules like:

'Be quiet.'

'Stay small.'

'Don't stand out.'

On trying not to stand out

'Don't stand out' was a big one for me (and many other women I know). For years I lived my life with the underlying belief that it was wrong to stand out. I kept myself quiet in groups. Even when I had an opinion on something and I could feel it bubbling away, dying to be expressed, I wouldn't speak up. I didn't realise at the time that it was taking *far* more energy to suppress what I wanted to say, than it would have done to actually express myself.

The number of times I sat in a group or a meeting with words literally on the tip of my tongue, but terrified of saying them out loud. The thought of saying the 'wrong thing' paralysed me. But, of course, I was assuming that whatever I had to say was the 'wrong thing'. Often I would hold back on saying something and someone else would say virtually the same thing a few minutes later. Then I would kick myself for not speaking up, using more and more energy as the internal dialogue in my head became louder and more critical. It would go something like this:

IGG: Nicola, keep quiet, it's too risky to say anything.

Me: But I really want to express myself. This view is just waiting to come out. I'm sure it would be okay?

IGG: No, you'll just make a fool of yourself. If you say something now, everyone will look at you and you'll just go red and feel stupid.

Me: But maybe I won't this time?

IGG: Who are you kidding? It's safer to keep your mouth shut. Then you can't get it wrong.

Then as someone piped up with the same thing I was going to say:

IGG: You really should have spoken up Nicola. There must be something wrong with you. Everyone else seems to be okay expressing themselves. Why can't you?

Me: Sigh.

Constantly self-monitoring and trying not to stand out in any way is exhausting.

Although I believed I was maintaining my identity as a good girl, keeping quiet was holding me back in lots of different ways. Particularly when I started to run my own business, I realised that if I wanted to be successful, I would have to stand out. A bland business doesn't attract clients, so I had to go through the uncomfortable process of showing more of myself. I gradually started to blog, record videos and share more of myself on social media.

And each step was challenging as my inner good girl would be there saying, 'No! Nicola, you can't show that. People will notice you.' In spite of this, I started to stretch my own internal rules and although it felt uncomfortable, each time I stretched my inner good girl became quieter and I connected more with my unbound self.

But I still like to sit in the right seat!

Take up space

The inner good girl has a tendency to shrink. Some of the self-imposed rules she sticks to are: 'Good girls don't stand out, don't make a fuss and don't impose on others', so the inner good girl figures it's best to make herself as small as possible.

How does this show up?

Physically making herself small – crossed legs, keeping her muscles tense, sitting with her legs tucked up underneath her.

Hovering on the edges of meetings, parties and events.

Sitting in corners.

Going to the back row.

Keeping quiet in meetings.

Wearing clothes that don't stand out.

All of these behaviours are designed to constrict and restrict, to keep oneself acceptable, inoffensive and, by definition, safe.

As I talked about above, I certainly used to feel more comfortable keeping myself super-small. I would rarely speak up in groups. Even if I was in a group of friends or family members, I would hold back on any impulse to speak and would keep quiet.

My underlying belief was, 'No-one wants to hear what I've got to say.' So I would hover on the outskirts or sit closed off and constricted, feeling tense and vulnerable. And, of course, if we feel closed off, tense and precarious, that's what gets reflected back to us by others.

I would leave meetings or workshops feeling frustrated that I hadn't shared what I'd wanted to, or irritated that someone else had chimed in with precisely the insight I wanted to share, but hadn't been brave enough to.

My mantra was, 'It's not safe to stand out', so I made very sure that I didn't. I shrunk myself to make others feel more comfortable, but of course, it just made me invisible.

I would only share something if I felt absolutely safe to do so. And it was exhausting, because I would constantly be monitoring myself.

Is it safe to say this?

Is it safe to do this?

Is it safe to wear this?

What will people think of me?

Over the years women have been encouraged to shrink away. Often women who put their heads seemingly above the parapet are shamed for doing so (and often by other women). We are impacted by centuries of cultural and societal conditioning to stay small.

The pink trousers

I remember a time during my counselling training when I was expanding my sense of self (much as you're doing now by reading this book) and I had just bought myself a pair of hot pink trousers. I usually wore fairly muted colours, so this was a departure for me. I had worn them for the first time and remember walking down the street feeling self-conscious, actually worrying that someone might make a critical comment about my pink slacks. (Seriously, I can't quite believe this now, but I was super-aware of how these trousers could make me stand out.)

I confided in one of the other women on my counselling course. She was an ex-punk and always dressed in the most beautiful, interesting, unusual clothes. I expected her to say, 'Fuck 'em! Just wear what you want and don't worry about what anyone else thinks.' But actually she advised me to be careful about where I chose to wear my pink trousers, suggesting that I could open myself up to criticism if I wore them in the 'wrong place'. She talked from years of experience and I felt deflated as I listened to her response.

Really? I had to be careful about where I chose to wear my pink trousers? My inner good girl certainly thought so, but my unbound self (who had taken a shine to the pink trousers in the first place) was despondent.

Now that I've worked with my inner good girl to let go of many self-imposed rules, I'm much more likely to wear the pink trousers without second-guessing. But I can still be wary of what I choose to wear, or taking up 'too much' space or attention. For example, I love to go bra-less. I love the feeling of freedom I get when I'm not wearing a bra and particularly in the summer, I'm often happy to go out sans bra. But I'll still be careful about where I go bra-less. God forbid that someone should spot one of my nipples through my clothes.

It's another inner good girl rule – 'Good girls keep themselves properly covered up'. They wear bras and they don't let their nipples show.

Jeez, my unbound self is super-frustrated by all of these perceived rules and limitations!

So how are you keeping yourself small at the moment? And what would it be like to take up more space?

Exercise – Experimenting with taking up space

We're going to keep it literal and physical with this exercise. Using your body and connecting with your physicality is one of the most powerful ways to create change.

1. Find a space where you have room to stand, sit and move freely. Tune into your inner good girl and imagine how she holds herself physically. Move into a position that represents your inner good girl.

   Notice how you feel in this position.

Is she moving or still?

Is she sitting, standing, reclining or something else?

How comfortable are you in this position?

Do you feel secure or precarious?

Would you be happy to stay in this position for a long time?

What parts of your body are you particularly aware of?

What happens to your energy in this position?

2. Now move out of your inner good girl position. Shake your body and shift position.

   Notice how it feels to move.

3. Tune into your unbound self and move yourself into a position that represents her.

Ask yourself the same questions as you did with your inner good girl position.

Take some time to journal on this experience. Write about how it felt to shift physically from your inner good girl into your unbound self.

Muscle memory is key. Now that you've tuned into your unbound self physically, you will be able to carry this into your everyday life.

And for more inspiration, check out the amazing Vanessa Kisuule and her video Take up Space on YouTube (www.youtube.com/watch?v=B72_O9D4jNg).

Exercise – Sticking to the rules

Do you like to stick to the rules? Where in your life is your inner good girl holding you back?

Spend 24 hours looking out for any internal rules you've set for yourself.

Notice the areas in your life where you're not fully being yourself because you're trying to play by the rules.

Who sets these rules? Where have they come from?

Where in your life could you start to stretch and bend the rules to be more you?

Experiment with challenging the rules you've set for yourself.

Give yourself permission to speak up and stand out. Notice how that feels.

Take some time to journal on your experience of sticking to the rules.

Online etiquette and the inner good girl

Remember the time when we didn't have email or even mobile phones? I do and it's not so long ago that the only way someone could contact you was by letter, landline or fax. But even if you can remember, it seems like a lifetime ago, doesn't it?

Now I'm not going to get all nostalgic and look back with rose-tinted glasses. I love the connectivity we have now. It's helped me to grow my business in a way that just wouldn't have been possible ten years ago. But with this increased ability to be in touch 24/7 come pressures and a new set of perceived rules to stick to. And, of course, as we've been talking about in this chapter, where there are rules to be followed, the inner good girl won't be far away.

With the rise of the internet, social media and mobile technology, each of us is more contactable than ever before and there are countless ways for others to get hold of us. (Mr H and I even communicate via online Scrabble sometimes when he's away!) You can be responding to email, replying to Facebook messages and checking what's happening on Instagram before you've even had breakfast.

But this increased connectivity can lead us to feel like we always need to respond instantly. Whereas in the past you may have spoken with a friend once a week on the phone, now there can be an endless back-and-forwards of WhatsApp messages. Maybe in the past you would have responded to new client enquiries once a day, but now you feel like you should get back to emails as soon as they appear in your inbox. Perhaps you spoke to your partner once (if at all) during the day when you were at work and now there can be numerous texts, flying between you whilst you're out of the house.

And this can help you to feel connected to those around you, which is obviously a wonderful thing, but it can often leave us feeling like we're permanently 'on' – on call and in demand. Remember all of those emails, messages and texts are taking place in addition to all the other stuff that fills our lives. No wonder we can often end up feeling overloaded and overwhelmed.

And the inner good girl is particularly susceptible to this need to be constantly in touch and available. Her need to please others and to stick to the rules means that if she receives an email, she wants to respond straight away. If she gets a voicemail that she can't respond to immediately, she'll send a text to explain why. She'll hastily reply to a Facebook message when she's in the cinema because she doesn't want to be seen to be rude.

She drives herself crazy trying to keep in touch and keep everyone happy. But when you always feel the need to respond instantly, you diminish your own needs. When you disrupt your schedule to get back to someone when it's not at all urgent, then you send a message to yourself and out into the Universe that 'I am not important. I don't value myself'.

Even when someone has an automatic email responder set up saying, 'I've received your email and will respond within the next 24 hours', I wonder why we even need to do this? Surely it's acceptable to allow one day to respond to messages? You don't need to justify how you spend your time or choose to respond to messages. Your unbound self knows this. And you can end up feeling completely scattered and ungrounded.

Now, I must admit that this is a work in progress for me. As I sit writing this, I've just posted a photo on Instagram and find myself checking my phone to see if there have been any comments or likes. As I see a comment, my first response is to reply immediately. My inner good girl is keen and pretty much wanting to do everything at once. But the truth is I've come to Southampton Central Library to write this afternoon, so I choose to honour the space I've created and to write. I have phases where I'll only check emails and Facebook twice a day and then slip back into constantly dipping online.

But an area where I am consistent is with my smartphone. Each night I turn it off completely at 9pm, so I can wind down and spend some 100% undisturbed time with Mr H. Even though my inner good girl pipes up with, 'What if someone wants to get hold of you?', I know it can always wait until morning. This is a non-negotiable, switch-off practice for me.

So, how about you? How do you feel about responding to messages and comments online? Do you feel under pressure to respond immediately? If so, why?

I invite you to reflect on this and to try out something different over the next few days.

Exercise – Online communication and boundaries

For the next 24 hours, designate one or two times during the day when you'll respond to messages (either online or via telephone). Decide when suits you and stick to it.

Notice any resistance and choose to move through it.

Affirm to yourself, 'My time is important and I choose when I'm available to others.'

If your inner good girl pipes up, send her some reassurance and let her know that you're experimenting with doing things differently.

Call on your unbound self to support you.

Notice how batching your online time impacts positively on your day.

Perhaps you feel more grounded, or centred or even (paradoxically) more connected?

How can you create some healthier boundaries around your online time and availability from now on?

What do you need to support yourself in doing this?

Write down your intentions.

STEP TEN – THE CULT OF BUSY-NESS AND SELF-CARE

One of the collective rules that we can get sucked into is a need to be busy – the cult of busy-ness.

The inner good girl loves to be seen as a productive member of society, so she will always find ways to keep herself busy.

When someone asks, 'How's things?', for many of us, the default response is, 'Great. Really busy. Lots going on.' We want people to know we've got it going on, we're needed, we're worthy.

'Can't stop.'

'Sorry, I'm in a rush!'

'It never stops, does it?'

'It's just one thing after another!'

'I just don't get a minute to myself.'

These statements can all be seen as complaints, but do we really wish it was different? Very often, they are presented as badges of honour. The truth is that in Western society, busy = good and quiet = well, a bit unsettling, unusual and, dare I say? Lazy.

Oh, that word, lazy. It strikes dread in the inner good girl. And I get this. I've had a huge fear of being seen as lazy in the past.

The life of Riley

When I left my corporate career and decided to retrain as a hypnotherapist, one of my main drivers was to create more freedom and flexibility for myself. I wanted more time for myself, more time to hang out with friends, to go out for lunch, have coffee dates, go to the forest or the beach for a walk, have fun.

The idea of flexibility over my time was so compelling after years in a 9–5 role. But, as I started my new business, I found I still felt the need to be seen as 'working' an 'acceptable' number of hours. The 9–5 mindset was still with me.

As he was going off to work in the morning, my husband would ask me what I had planned for the day and my inner good girl would immediately slip into defence mode. 'I'm working' I would say and reel off a list of tasks I was going to do and client appointments. I felt the need to demonstrate the busy-ness in my business.

If I ever had something other than 'work' planned, like a walk on the beach or lunch with a friend, Mr H would often respond with 'Oh, you're living the life of Riley!' and my inner good girl would take this as an insult, an insinuation that I was lazy.

This went on for a long time, my need to defend my reputation as a productive and certainly non-lazy member of society. Until one day after a 'life of Riley' comment in the morning, I was out for a walk on the beach and something clicked within me. My unbound self thought, 'Hang on. I've chosen to create this life for myself. I've chosen to leave the corporate world. I've taken a risk and decided to start my own business because I want more freedom and flexibility. *What if there's nothing actually wrong with living the life of Riley?'*

What if I just stopped feeling the need to defend myself?

What if I let go of the need to prove my 'busy-ness'?

What if I just said, 'Yep. I am living the life of Riley because that's what I've chosen to do.'

The idea was exhilarating. As I look back, I can see that my unbound self was completely in play here. She was in her element – on the beach, feeling free – and she decided to make a direct challenge to my inner good girl.

In that moment, I decided that it was okay to take time out. It was okay to meet a friend for coffee, to go to the spa or take myself off for a walk in a nature, when in the past I might have felt like I 'should' be working.

It was okay to rest, to take a nap in the afternoon and just do nothing.

My unbound self was pushing against the collective cult of busy-ness. And I felt liberated. I remember driving home from the beach and embracing my new commitment to the life of Riley.

And now when Mr H asks what I'm doing that day, I feel much more comfortable with answering honestly, not feeling that I need to come up with a list of productive tasks (although my inner good girl still gets defensive sometimes).

This need to be busy, this collective rule, is endemic though, particularly amongst women. So many clients I've worked with have struggled with feeling lazy or self-indulgent if they dare to make time for themselves.

When I surveyed my community, 37% said they often like to be seen as productive and create tasks to keep themselves busy. Some of the examples given were:

Having time to just 'be' is time wasted – I should be tidying, cleaning, checking in on friends, etc.

I realise I used to do this all the time to justify my existence, particularly when I was 'only a housewife and mother' with an enormous house to decorate and run and 3 children and a business! I am learning now that time out is not only essential but that doing things for their own sake is good too, and pleasure is gooooood!

I knit; sew; bake; do online courses, projects to keep me busy and show I am a good girl using my time productively, yet I spend a lot of time just browsing the internet so that I don't have to engage with my own thoughts.

My to-do list is always 2 or 3 pages long and if it's shorter I sit down and mind map new projects and fill up the to do list again.

There seems to be this collective fear of letting go and stopping. Because who are you when you're doing nothing? We tend to define ourselves through activity. When we meet someone new, very often one of the first questions we ask or get asked is, 'So, what do you do?' And the inner good girl feels comfortable with this question. It allows her to give a clear, concise, socially acceptable answer.

What about being?

Lessons from a burn-out

In the summer of 2015 I felt burned out in my business. I was tired and totally lacking in motivation. I could barely get myself off the sofa. And apart from actually seeing my clients, every other element of my business took a back seat.

I stopped blogging.

I stopped posting on social media.

I stopped sending my weekly newsletter.

My creative well was dry.

I knew I needed to rest. I actually couldn't do anything else.

So I did. I slept and laid and dozed and watched TV and went for gentle walks.

And a magical thing happened.

The world didn't stop.

I found I still had enough clients.

I still made enough money.

Even though I wasn't rushing around being 'productive', I was okay and I was supported.

I called this my period of radical non-action and I now encourage my clients to (non) do this too – to take some time to simply be, to rest, to step back and reflect on the perceived need to 'do'. Maybe you could too?

Potent decluttering

Decluttering is a buzzword right now. There are books, blogs and workshops all devoted to the art of decluttering.

So, here's another definition for you.

Decluttering: to remove unnecessary items from (an untidy and overcrowded place).

Much of the content out there is focused on physical decluttering – letting go of possessions that you no longer need and want. Physical decluttering is very powerful. When you have a physical clear-out, you naturally make space for the new to flow in.

However, emotional and energetic decluttering is just as important. And it goes hand-in-hand with physical decluttering.

What do I mean by emotional and energetic decluttering? I see this as letting go of any beliefs, relationships, obligations, commitments or tasks that no longer serve us. As you've been working through this book, you will naturally have been doing this kind of decluttering, as you've started to change old beliefs and patterns. And now it's time to move onto a new area of letting go.

As I've mentioned the inner good girl loves to be seen as busy. It's one of her internal rules – I must keep busy. She also likes to please others. And this can be deadly combination, as she will tend to hold on to a whole host of situations, commitments and 'to-dos' that are not necessarily in her best interests.

I'm on a continual process of decluttering and every so often I take a step back to review what I've got going on in my life.

What's taking up my time?

Who am I spending time with?

What am I focusing on?

What's on my to-do list?

And does all of this still serve me?

In her fantastic book on decluttering, *The Life-Changing Magic of Tidying*, Marie Kondo advises you to ask one question when deciding whether to keep hold of possessions – 'Does this spark joy?'

I love this question. It cuts through the 'shoulds' and the 'musts' and the 'ought tos' (all of the downfalls of the inner good girl). 'Does it spark joy?' gets to the crux of how we feel, which is always the most powerful way to make decisions.

You know instantly if something sparks joy in you, or not. You can feel it in your body (even if you try and kid yourself). And you can use exactly the same question when you're making decisions about whether to keep or let go of commitments, clients, tasks, relationships, situations and activities. This one simple question is like magic.

In this epidemic of busy-ness, decluttering your commitments is vital. Do you really need to be rushing around from one place to another, never getting time to be you?

No.

I wager you could let go of between 50% and 80% of your current activities and everything would be okay. I know that might sound very unlikely to the inner good girl, but it's the truth. I've seen it personally and with clients.

So, in this stage of the process, I'm asking you to step back and reflect on your current schedule. How are you choosing to fill your time?

Exercise – Does it spark joy? Making space for your unbound self

Get out your diary or calendar and write down every activity you do during an average week. Add to the list any other regular activities or events you can think of.

You'll likely end up with a pretty long list and that's okay.

Take a deep breath and set your intention.

'I choose to make space for my unbound self.'

Now go through each item on the list and ask, 'Does this spark joy?'

Notice what answer comes to mind. Don't rush this. Pay attention to how you feel in your body.

As you look at each item on the list, do you feel expansive or constricted? (You can't fool your body. Just as we did with good girl goals, your body will let you know if an activity is draining you, rather than filling you up.)

'Does it spark joy?'

When you're finished, notice how many items on your list really do spark joy. It's likely to be between 20% and 50%. If it's not you've probably done some potent decluttering before.

What would it be like to let go of anything on your list that doesn't truly spark joy?

Freeing?

Exciting?

Scary?

I get it. The inner good girl likes to stick to her commitments (even if they're self-imposed). But this process is all about making more space for the unbound self.

So, what could you easily let go of?

There will be some items on your list you could let go of in a second. Easy peasy.

Do it. Let go of the easy stuff.

Maybe the Facebook group that drags you down every time you see notifications, or the magazine subscription you never get around to reading, or the gym class you're always putting off.

Let it go.

Then you can move on to anything that feels more challenging. Know that you are making more space for the stuff that lights you up.

Here are some time commitments that I've decluttered in the past:

- Being the Group Leader of a networking group.
- Online memberships.
- Non-ideal clients.
- Regular client work on a retreat that involved too much travel.
- Facebook groups I had started and then fallen out of love with.
- Business ideas that weren't in alignment with my desires.

All of this allowed me to have more space to do the things I love. And to not do.

At times I procrastinated on making these decisions. My inner good girl worried, 'What will people think of me?', 'What if I upset that person?', 'What if they think I'm a flake?' or 'What if letting go of this means I'll never attract another good opportunity ever again?'

All of those fears were ungrounded.

When you let go of something, when you say, 'Actually, I've chosen not to do this any more', you give others permission to do the same. In making space for yourself, you allow others to do the same. It's a powerful ripple effect.

When I took a client through this exercise recently, that's exactly what happened. She was feeling drained and wanted to make self-care a priority.

When we looked at how she was spending her time, she could see that she had been spending up to ten hours a week doing voluntary work for a charity she was involved in. Now this charity was important to her, but she had her own business to run, a family to look after and self-care to fit in too. She had been doing bits and pieces of work for the charity spread throughout the week whenever she had time. If something came up and she knew she could do it, she would, even if it didn't fit within her role.

I asked how much time she wanted to spend on her charity work each week and she answered that three hours per week would feel good. I suggested that she boundary the time she spent on this charity work and batch her three hours together on one day.

Obviously it was quite a big shift to move from ten hours per week to three, so I asked her to experiment with the new arrangement and see how it went.

Hint: When you approach a change as an experiment, rather than something that's set in stone, it takes the pressure off and your inner good girl is more likely to go along with it.

When I spoke to my client the following week, she was amazed at how easy it had been to reduce and boundary the hours she was spending on her charity work. And when she spoke to a colleague about it, her fellow charity worker decided to do the same thing. She gave this other woman permission to make more space for herself too.

When you look at it like this, letting go or reducing commitments that drain you is anything but selfish. Often you will inspire others to do the same.

Here's to breaking those self-imposed rules and living a more unbound life!

STEP ELEVEN – ANGER AND EXPRESSING EMOTION

Every inner good girl is different. Every inner good girl has her own characteristics and quirks. Yours is as unique as you are. But something that many inner good girls have in common is the belief that it's wrong to express anger.

When asked whether they agreed with the statement, 'I don't like to express anger and often suppress my feelings, rather than creating conflict', 47% of respondents said they did this often or all the time.

Some of the examples were:

I absolutely hate conflict and will do almost anything to avoid having to deal with difficult people or have uncomfortable conversations. Again this is an area that I am working on – that it is ok to speak my mind and to disagree or to state my feelings on something.

Absolutely. I don't say what's on my mind if something has hurt me or angered me. When I do get angry I cry which is very frustrating.

I find it very hard to say what I think so I am considered a nice person, always willing to help. I want to scream leave me alone. I once worked with a person who was very manipulative and eventually caused me to leave my job but I could never say anything against her as in my mind it would seem as if it was sour grapes.

I hate conflict. It makes me nauseous and anxious.

Pretty much every one of us was told off as a child for getting angry. If you weren't directly told off, then it's likely that those around you implied in some way that anger was bad. So we learned to hold it in.

And of course anger is a perfectly natural emotion, like all of the others. But it seems to have been singled out for almost universal condemnation.

Parents don't like anger.

Teachers don't like anger.

Society doesn't like anger.

In fact, any strong emotion tends to be frowned upon.

The process I'm guiding you through here is designed to help you connect and express all the different, complex aspects of you. Your unbound self is a full expression of these aspects. And the inner good girl is only able to express those parts of you (and those emotions) that are deemed to be acceptable. Somewhere along the line your inner good girl learned that certain emotions are inherently bad.

As I mentioned earlier, throughout my life I've always been seen as a calm person. I've often been praised for this quality and as I've grown older, it's kinda bugged me. As I've come to do this healing work, I've realised that the reason it bugs me is that I have a whole heap of unexpressed 'stuff' bubbling away within me.

My mask

When I was little I remember having a dream. I'm not sure exactly how old I was, but I was very young, around six or seven years old.

In the dream I was lying on some kind of bed in a clinical-looking room; it may have been an operating theatre. Someone came in and placed a mask over my face; it was a completely blank, white, plaster mask. It had no breathing holes or space for the mouth. It covered my face entirely.

I still remember now the feeling as that mask was placed on my face. I was terrified. It felt stifling, like I couldn't breathe. And the mask felt heavy and restrictive.

I can still remember that dream vividly even now. It seems like a very strange dream for a young girl to have. But as I reflect on it, I can see that it represents the mask I wore for a large part of my life, up until my late thirties.

The mask of someone who is calm and happy and easy-going. And although I didn't always realise that I was wearing a mask, it was stifling. That mask was stifling the real me – my unbound self.

> *'Lift the masks, remove the armour and let yourself become all that imagined.'*
> *Flavia*

Even after doing my hypnotherapy and counselling training and the personal therapy that comes with that, for a long time, I didn't know exactly what I had been masking, the feelings that had been unexpressed. I worked through all the usual suspects – guilt, shame, sadness, fear – but I could still feel a tension in the pit of my stomach. I can feel it now as I write and I've only recently realised what it is – anger. In fact, it feels closer to rage.

When I connected with my unbound self, I was surprised at just how wild and dark she was. In fact, I was a bit disappointed. I imagined that my unbound self would be joyful and playful – all of the lovely 'acceptable' qualities I thought I wanted more of in my life. But here was this witchy, powerful, rage-filled being. And she scared me.

Now that I've had more time to process it, I realise that it makes perfect sense. Of course, my unbound self will hold all of those qualities and emotions I've held down and felt unable to express in the past. So, as I've always been comfortable showing the light, 'nice' parts of myself, the unbound me will have a larger proportion of the dark, 'not nice' stuff.

And the bit I've been most unable to express throughout my life has been anger. So it's built up and built up, at times erupting in moments of lashing out, but mostly held down.

And I'm not alone in this, as the respondents of my survey confirm. Over the years I've worked with many clients who are good girls on the surface – nice and calm and accommodating to their friends and families – but when we start working, there is an anger, a rage bubbling away underneath.

What happens to all of that anger?

What happens to all the anger women hold in and put a firm lid on?

It turns in on you.

It drains your energy.

It becomes toxic.

It manifests physically as pain, illness or disease.

It manifests in destructive relationships.

It manifests in unfulfilled dreams.

The anger is often related to unexpressed desires, a feeling of powerlessness (more on this in the next chapter). So, rather than masking it and carrying on regardless, it's helpful to uncover what your anger is trying to tell you.

Exercise – Listening to your anger

Although I'm talking specifically about anger here, this exercise can be used to tune into any emotion and discover the message it has for you.

Why is this important?

Well, our emotions are a powerful guidance system; they let us know if we're going in the right direction. So, if you're feeling joyful, loving or peaceful (for example), you can be pretty sure you're on track in that moment. However, if you're feeling stressed, or frustrated or angry, then it's likely that something is off-kilter.

Rather than suppressing those uncomfortable emotions (the feelings that are often deemed to be unacceptable by the inner good girl), we need to listen to what they're telling us. This is what this exercise has been designed to do.

Hint: I suggest doing this exercise even if you don't feel particularly angry at the moment. In fact, it can be especially helpful in this case. At times when you're actually aware of your anger, when it's up on the surface, it's likely that you have a pretty good idea of what's caused it. However, when we have an active inner good girl, it's very possible that any anger you're experiencing is hidden and out of your awareness. If you feel that you never get angry or know that you feel uncomfortable expressing anger, then this exercise will be particularly helpful for you.

Don't forget, you can download a free MP3 of this exercise on the link below:
www.nicolahumber.com/heal-your-inner-good-girl-bonuses

1. Take a moment, somewhere quiet, and make yourself comfortable, either sitting or lying down.

2. Close your eyes and take three deep breaths, breathing right down into your belly with a wonderful, releasing breath out each time.

3. Allow your breath to settle and bring your attention into your body; just notice how you feel physically in this moment.

4. Ask yourself (silently in your mind), where in my body am I holding anger?

5. Notice which part of your body you feel drawn to as you ask this question. Is it your stomach, your chest, your throat, or somewhere else? (As with many of the previous exercises, be open to whatever comes to you. Allow yourself to be guided by your body and your subconscious mind.)

6. Take your attention to the part of your body where you're holding anger and notice how you experience it physically. What sensations are you aware of? Does it feel tight or scattered? Heavy or light? Hot or cold? Moving or still? What does this feeling remind you of?

7. What colour is this feeling? Notice what colour comes to mind, even if it feels like you're making it up.

8. As you remain focused on all of the qualities of this feeling – where you're holding it in your body, how you experience it physically and its colour – ask yourself, 'What do you need me to know?'

9. As you ask this question, notice what comes to mind. It may be a memory, an image, a statement or even one word. It may just be a sense of something. Or perhaps your unbound self will come into your awareness with a message for you? As always, choose to be open to whatever comes, without judgement.

10. Spend a few more moments relaxing and giving space to whatever needs to come. It's possible that you may feel emotion rising to the surface and that's okay. Just allow it to come and be released.

11. When you're ready, open your eyes and take some time to journal on

whatever came up for you during the exercise. Write about any insights you gained, any messages you received. What was it like to give a voice to that feeling that you usually push down?

The point of this exercise is not to discover what's made you angry and go vent at that person or situation. We're not looking to direct our anger outwards into the world. The aim is to harness the power of your anger and to channel that in a helpful way, rather than suppressing it.

Simply by doing this exercise, you have given more space to an emotion that maybe you haven't even been able to acknowledge in the past.

Then again, maybe you've been only too aware that there was anger bubbling away within you because at times it erupts like a volcano of shouting, screaming and even physical violence? Because the inner good girl has a tendency to hold anger in at any cost, when it eventually rises to the surface, it can seem out of proportion and explosive.

By not giving a voice to our anger, it becomes out of our control.

I've certainly experienced this in the past. As it was part of my identity to be seen as calm, any anger I experienced was held in and pushed down. If I felt in conflict with someone, I would bite my tongue and try and keep the peace. But, of course, this isn't sustainable.

So, every now and again my anger would explode. Often it would be directed at someone I was close to, usually my sister or a partner. And when this happened, it would feel uncontrollable.

I remember at least two of these times when I've slapped my sister across the face during one of these outbursts. And I'm pretty sure I wasn't even angry with her at these times. Our argument and me lashing out was a manifestation of the anger I had been suppressing for so long, the part of me I hadn't been expressing.

I feel so ashamed that I slapped my sister. As I look back, I can't quite believe that I did it. It's almost like I became someone else in those moments.

And when I was speaking to other women about anger during the writing of this book, many had had similar experiences.

One time when I was at a networking group, I mentioned that I was writing about anger and asked to speak to angry women. When I announced this in front of the whole group, no-one said anything. So, I thought, 'Well, maybe it's just me who experiences this?'

But at the break, one woman after another came up and took me to one side to confess that she was an 'angry woman'. Many of them had tales of uncontrollable outbursts followed by shame and guilt.

It's such a toxic cycle. The inner good girl causes us to keep our anger hidden and when it does inevitably explode, she makes us feel guilty and ashamed for exposing what she sees to be an unacceptable side of us.

Sometimes my anger explosions would be directed at myself. I would have episodes where I felt hopeless and ugly. My inner critical voice would turn on me and say things like: 'What's wrong with you? You can't get anything right. You're pathetic. What's the point of you being here?'

These were very low points and although I didn't self-harm, I can certainly imagine that this might have happened at times like this. When anger is turned inwards like this, it's poisonous. But for many women, it feels like the only option. Because the inner good girl is so adamant that anger should not be shown to the outside world.

After doing the last exercise, you will have begun to tap into the message that any anger you're experiencing has for you. This in itself is a powerful release. And now I invite you to think about different ways you could choose to express your anger, without directing it at someone else or back in at yourself.

When I first connected with my unbound self and saw how rage-filled she was, I knew that I had to do something to release the intense anger that had built up within me without me being aware of it. First of all, I wrote about it. I turned to a fresh page in my journal and began to write about all the things I felt angry about. It was difficult to tap into this at first, but as I wrote the words began to come more and more easily.

I'm angry at……

I'm angry at……

I'm angry at…..

I could feel the energy building up within me as I wrote quicker and quicker, and then something shifted and the energy subsided again. I knew that by writing the words, by choosing to acknowledge all the things I had been angry at and never expressed, a powerful release had occurred.

After this initial journaling, I had a sense that I needed to do something more physical to release any anger that might build up from then on. Inspired by my unbound self, one of my words for 2016 was 'fierce', so I decided to sign up for a kung fu class to give an outlet for my fierceness.

I had never done any form of martial arts before (apart from the gentle practice of tai chi), so kung fu felt very new for me. But it was exhilarating to learn how to punch and kick, to be encouraged to hit as hard as I could, to channel the aggression within me.

To be honest, at times I find kung fu challenging, as I'm tapping into a part of myself that I've only recently uncovered. However, I feel very different now that I have a particular way to express my anger physically. I feel like I have more energy generally, because the truth is it saps a huge amount of energy when you're trying to hold emotions in. When you find a resourceful way to express your emotions, it frees up energy within you.

So, how will you choose to express your anger (or any other heavier emotions that your inner good girl has encouraged you to keep hidden in the past)?

Here are some ideas for you:

- Journal on it. Just as I did, ask yourself, 'What am I angry at?' and begin to write. The words will begin to flow very quickly.
- Write a letter to anyone or anything you feel angry towards. This is not a letter to be sent. It's purely for you to express how you're feeling onto the page.
- Go to a boxing or martial arts class.
- Have a regular cardio workout.
- Dance it out – put on your favourite angry music and go for it!
- Shout it out – find somewhere you can shout or scream and let your rage out that way.
- Paint your anger – get a piece of paper or a canvas and express your emotions visually onto the page.
- Go for a run or vigorous walk. Combining being outside with movement is very healing, so take yourself for a run or walk and use this as a way to release any anger that's built up.

These are just some ideas and you may well have another way that you want to express any pent-up emotion. The important thing is to do this regularly. Make it a regular practice.

All emotions are meant to move. They are not meant to be stagnant and suppressed. So any way you can find to release them will create a huge shift in the way you feel on a day-to-day basis.

STEP TWELVE – KNOWING WHAT YOU WANT AND LIVING AN UNBOUND LIFE

The inner good girl will often encourage you to keep your desires hidden. However small they may be, asking for what you want seems risky to the inner good girl.

Maybe your desires are unreasonable?

Maybe your desires are unusual?

Maybe asking for what you want will put someone else out?

Maybe stating your desires will make someone angry?

In any case, being clear about what you want could well mean that the other people in your life (your partner, friend, children, parents, colleagues) may not be able to get their full needs met. And for the inner good girl, that is not okay.

As you've seen throughout this book, one of her mottos is 'Don't make a fuss', which basically means, 'Don't put anyone out'. And asking for what you want is very much seen as making a fuss by the inner good girl. So she fits in. When someone asks what she wants to do, her default response is, 'I don't mind, you choose.'

Nothing too wrong about that, is there? She goes with the flow. What a 'good' trait to have. But there is a hidden danger of going with the flow.

When we don't acknowledge and express what we want, our desires get pushed down. They can become hidden, even from ourselves. We forget what it is that we actually want. We tell ourselves, I don't feel strongly about that. And when we lose track of our desires, we begin to lose our sense of self.

With the Law of Attraction and particularly in the teachings of Abraham Hicks, it's our desires that create our world. Our desires help us to expand our world. And without them, we become rudderless. We drift and float in a sea of 'I don't mind', 'You choose' and 'I'm happy to go with the flow'.

I worked with a client once who had totally lost track of herself. She told me that when she went for a meal with her husband, it had got to the point where he would choose from the menu for her, not because he was controlling, but because she had no clue what she wanted.

She had lost her sense of self.

She had been trying to please everyone – her parents, her husband, her friends, her children – her whole life and now she couldn't even decide what main course she would like. So when it came to bigger decisions, decisions that would truly shape her world, she was in despair, so confused that she couldn't see a way forward.

And the scary thing is that I could identify with her. Even with all the personal development work I've done over the years, I'm still not clear on what I truly want at times. Often I find myself saying, 'I don't mind' when my husband asks me where I want to spend the evening. And okay, sometimes it's not hugely important, but every time we say, 'I don't mind' it sends a message to ourselves and out into the world that we don't really matter.

When I asked my community whether they identified with the statement – 'Sometimes I find it difficult to know what I really want, because I tend to go along with what those around me choose' – over a quarter said often or all the time.

Here are some of the examples given:

My husband asks me what I would like to do for my birthday, and I find it so hard to decide. I wish he would just surprise me, because thinking what I really want is so difficult for me!

Trying to gain a consensus for celebrating my birthday to keep everyone happy rather than choosing exactly what I want.

Eek!!! I find it very, very difficult to choose what I really want and often feel like I just want to 'fit in'. I remember being asked what I wanted from my life and I found it really difficult to answer!!! Even choosing a restaurant to go to is not easy for me!!!

If asked what I want to do I ask the question back, and then fit in with them rather than say well I would like to do... I have noticed that on the occasions when I do speak up it is never what the consensus go with so why bother speaking in the first place?

I spoke about this with my mum recently. We were on a day trip to Bath with my sister and before getting the train, we went to get a coffee. When the barista asked my mum what milk she would prefer, she said, 'Oh, I don't mind.' The barista asked again, 'No, it's fine. What would you like?' And my mum said, 'Skimmed if you've got it, but it doesn't matter if not.' When she saw that the barista would have to open a new carton of skimmed milk, Mum quickly jumped in with a 'Don't worry if you have to open a new one, I'll have whatever you've got.'

Sigh.

Like many women (and particularly mothers), my beautiful mum tends to put other people's needs above her own. She is a real 'I don't mind. You choose' kinda gal. And as I was writing this chapter, the experience in the coffee shop really stood out for me. I brought it up with Mum later over lunch. I asked why she found it difficult to ask for what she wanted.

Mum argued that when it comes to bigger issues, she will make her desires known, but with small things (like what milk to have in her coffee), she can't see the point. It doesn't really matter and she's happy to go with the flow.

I understand this and I felt the same for many years (probably because I saw this so often from Mum when growing up). But as I wrote earlier, every time we say 'I don't mind' it sends a message to ourselves and out into the Universe that we're not important.

The unbound self never says, 'I don't mind.' She expresses her desires, her wants, clearly. She knows what she wants.

Your desires shape your world. They give it colour, texture, detail. Your desires are clues to who you truly are. They are important.

What do you prefer?

Where do you like to go?

How do you like to spend your time?

Who lights you up?

What's your favourite meal?

What would you choose to do right now if you could?

What do you love wearing?

However insignificant the answers to these questions might feel, each one signposts you to where you truly want to be, to who you are.

The inner good girl prefers bland, nice, easy choices. But by fitting in and saying, 'I don't mind' you not only lose track of your true self, but your unexpressed desires get pushed down and become toxic. Even if you're not aware of them bubbling away deep within you, all of those unexpressed wants are there. They can turn into anger, rage and despair. And as I talked about in the last chapter, they will come out at some point.

Exercise – The 'I don't mind' diet

For the next 24 hours (at least), saying the words 'I don't mind' is NOT an option for you.

Whenever someone gives you a choice, make a decision.

If a friend asks you where you want to go for lunch, choose.

If your partner asks you what you want to watch on TV, choose.

If someone asks you how you would like to celebrate your birthday or another occasion, choose.

It doesn't matter if you don't feel strongly or you don't really know what you would like to do, just make a decision and choose.

Don't worry about getting it 'right', 'making a fuss' or putting the other person out. Just choose.

Notice any resistance to this and if your inner good girl chimes in with a 'Just go with the flow. It's easier', let her know that you're trying something different and that your choices are important.

Although you may feel that you don't have any real preference at first, by verbalising your choices, you're allowing your desires to bubble to the surface.

Notice how you feel physically, mentally and emotionally to be the one who decides. Take some time to journal on your experiences afterwards and resolve to make more definite choices from now on.

An unbound life

By now, you've got a clear idea of where your inner good girl has been impacting on your life; you've got to understand that part of you better and form a more resourceful relationship with her, as you've also begun to connect with your unbound self.

You've done a lot!

But it's possible you're still confused. Perhaps you're thinking, 'I thought the idea of this book was to ditch my inner good girl and 100% embrace my unbound self?' And in reality you've begun to develop a more compassionate relationship with your inner good girl. It's possible now that you actually feel quite loving towards her. In fact, I hope you do.

Maybe you still feel more comfortable with your inner good girl than your unbound self?

For many years, you've been living under the guidance of your inner good girl.

Her ideas are likely to seem very familiar to you. Whereas your unbound self may feel a bit 'out there'. Remember, though, both your inner good girl and unbound self are parts of you. So even if your unbound self seems completely unfamiliar, she's come from within you. She represents a freer, more authentic expression of you. And like all the different parts of you, she has your best interests at heart.

So, it's time to start listening to your unbound self a bit more and think about what an unbound life would look like for you.

The simplest way to do this is to look back through the notes you've made as you've been reading this book and focus on the areas of your life where you felt your inner good girl was restricting you in some way. The very fact that you've felt limited in these areas gives you a powerful clue as to where your unbound self could come into play.

If you felt your inner good girl showing up in your relationships, then how could you tap into your unbound self more in this area? Maybe you want to reevaluate what you say 'Yes' and 'No' to in future? Perhaps you want to reflect on your current goals and make some changes here?

The fact is your unbound self can put a whole new slant on everything, and that could feel overwhelming (understandably!). So it's best to take this step-by-step.

> '*It is by tiny steps we ascend to the stars.*'
> Jack Ludstrom

You can start by looking at the area of your life where your inner good girl was having the most impact. Whether it's your work, relationships, health or something else, this is the place to bring in your unbound self first.

And it's really quite simple to do this. Just ask yourself the question, 'What would my unbound self do here?'

This is going to be a power question for you from now on. (*Hint: You'll be using it a LOT!*)

You can either ask it during meditation and notice what insights come to you, or you can journal on it, or just ask it in the moment when you have a new opportunity, idea or situation presented to you.

We've been working with the subconscious mind throughout this process and by asking your power question, you are accessing this internal wisdom once again. Whenever you ask yourself a question, your subconscious mind can't help but find an answer. It may not come straight away, but you can know that your subconscious is looking for the answer and will present it to you at some point. Maybe when you're out for a walk or in the shower, an insight will pop into your head and that's your subconscious answering your question.

'What would my unbound self do here?'

Notice how you feel when you ask this question. It's likely that you'll notice a sense of expansion, an opening, excitement. When this happens, you know that you're tapping into that limitless part of you, the part of you that believes that anything is possible.

Once you have your answer, it's time to start taking action.

If you're struggling with promoting yourself, maybe your unbound self would do more public speaking?

If you're feeling stifled in a relationship, perhaps your unbound self would prefer to be alone?

If you're feeling stuck and unappreciated in a job, your unbound self might start her own business?

The truth is that your unbound self is likely to think big. She probably won't be interested in small manageable steps. So her answers may well strike you with fear initially. And that's okay. It's completely natural to feel apprehensive about making big changes (and the shift between listening to your inner good girl and tuning into your unbound self could be massive).

Know that you don't have to do it all at once. Your unbound self is at one end of the spectrum and your inner good girl is at the other. The aim of this process is to become more flexible in moving along it.

Remember, it's always your choice. Sometimes you might choose to roll with your inner good girl, especially now you've helped her do some healing. You might choose to keep the status quo for a while, particularly at times when your life is feeling chaotic.

Other times you'll be feeling like you can take on the world and you're ready to follow your unbound self 100% – new career, new relationship, world travels. Bring it on!

And other times, you're likely to be somewhere in-between, edging towards your unbound self, making incremental, expansive changes which are opening you up to a place of possibility.

The important words to remember here are 'choice' and 'expansion'. Always know that you have a choice. You're in the driving seat of your life, not anyone else or even one particular part of you. You get to decide what to do (or not do).

Also know that a feeling of expansion is likely to be leading you in the right direction. If thinking about something makes you feel more open and expansive, then you can be pretty sure it will be good for you.

But always know that you can't get this wrong.

I always encourage my clients to see life as a playful experiment. If something doesn't work out, you can always decide to do something different. We all know that nothing is permanent. The nature of the world is change. So, no decision is forever. And that feels pretty freeing, doesn't it?

Just try things out. Let go of specific expectations and see where your unbound self leads you.

Here are some suggestions to connect with your unbound self:

Take a different route.

Go on a journey alone.

Dance.

Sing.

Journal.

Get messy.

Draw.

Create.

Take a nap in the middle of the day.

Say yes.

Say no.

Speak up.

Dress down.

Dress up.

Wear a different colour.

Just be.

Do something indulgent, just for you.

Play.

Lie on the earth and look up at the sky.

Stretch.

Go first.

Breathe deep.

Take the day off.

Swim in the sea.

Walk barefoot.

Change your appearance.

Go slow.

These are just some of the possibilities. See what calls to you and always check in with your intention. Are you trying to do the 'right thing' and be a good girl? Or are you tapping into your unbound self?

Here's to living your unbound life!

AFTERWORD

As I came to the end of writing this book, my first book, my much-longed-for book, I felt a sense of dread and fear.

I talked to my accountability buddy, Jess, about it. She's writing her first book too and we speak each week on Skype, checking in, motivating each other and supporting each other through any resistance. I mentioned that I was struggling with how to end the book. I had no idea how to finish it, so I was feeling stuck.

Jess talked me through my stuck-ness and reassured me that it was natural to feel like this as I came closer to putting my work out into the world. As we spoke, I realised that I often felt this way about endings. Whenever I've come to the end of something – a job, a relationship, a course – I've preferred to slip away quietly, not celebrating or even acknowledging the ending and moving quickly onto the next 'thing'.

And of course, this is a tendency of my inner good girl. She hates to make a fuss and endings normally involve receiving attention of some kind (either positive or negative), so she steers clear and tries to avoid them.

So as I came towards the end of writing this book, a process that has taken seven months, I could feel my inner good girl's resistance coming up. But it felt like more than wanting to avoid 'the fuss' of an ending.

One evening recently, I mentioned my resistance to Mr H over dinner and he nailed it with his insight. (Much as it pains me to admit it, Mr H is quite the wise soul.) He suggested that my resistance was fear of having exactly the same kind of experience that had crystallised my inner good girl in the first place – taking my work up to the teacher and having it rubbished.

Ah, yes! That was it.

My stuck-ness wasn't just about endings; it was a deep terror of presenting my treasured work to the world and receiving a negative response. What if the world turned around and said 'Well, Nicola has just published her book and it's absolute rubbish!'

And maybe this is what has stopped me from writing a book before? It's been an ambition of mine for as long as I can remember. I've started to write different books and then tailed off. In fact, I've often found it challenging to finish projects. I'm all about the idea, the planning and getting started, but finishing? I rarely make it to the finish.

As I had this discussion with Mr H, I realised that my inner good girl was scared of being hurt, of being shamed, of being criticised, so in the past she had often prevented me from putting myself out there by actually finishing what I had started. Talking about this fear and bringing it out into the open helped to create a shift within me.

I chose to decide that what I had written was good enough.

Finishing and releasing this book into the world is a huge part of the healing process for my inner good girl. I want her to know that it's okay to speak up, it's okay to share yourself, it's okay to get it wrong or get it right, to not be perfect or to be perfect in your glorious imperfection. It's okay to write a book just because you want to and if someone else enjoys it or finds your words helpful, then that's a bonus.

So, as I write these last words, I feel some emotion rising to the surface and a sense of tenderness towards my inner good girl that wasn't there at the beginning of this journey.

How does my unbound self feel about finishing this book and putting it 'out there'? 'Fuck it Nic, stop over-thinking and just do it! Once this is done, something new begins.'

You've gotta love your unbound self, eh?

And for you? I send you my hope that this process has shifted something within you. I hope it's given you a greater understanding and compassion towards your inner good girl. And I hope it's helped you connect more with your very own unbound self.

I send love to each and every unique part of YOU.

Happy travels my friend!

Nicola x

CONTINUE THE JOURNEY

Nicola invites you to continue the Heal Your Inner Good Girl journey by joining her in the Unbound Living Group over on Facebook.

Head on over to the link below to join and become part of the Unbound Living community of women, committed to being their fullest, most brilliant selves!

www.facebook.com/groups/unboundwithnicolahumber

Don't forget to download your free Heal Your Inner Good Girl resources and bonuses by signing-up on the link below:

www.nicolahumber.com/heal-your-inner-good-girl-bonuses/

RECOMMENDED READING

'The Desire Map. A Guide to Creating Goals with Soul' by Danielle Laporte

'Succulent Wild Woman. Dancing With Your Wonder-full Self!' by SARK

'When the Body Says No. Exploring the Stress-Disease Connection' by Gabor Mate M.D.

'The Big Leap' by Gay Hendricks Ph.D.

'Big Magic. Creative Living, Beyond Fear' by Elizabeth Gilbert

'Lean In. Women, Work and the Will to Lead' by Sheryl Sandberg

'The Life-Changing Magic of Tidying' by Marie Kondo

'Ask and it is Given' by Esther and Jerry Hicks

ACKNOWLEDGEMENTS

To Cathy and Chris Semple. For encouraging, supporting and accepting me through all the twisty, turny choices I've made in my life.

To Louise Semple. For being my soul sister. For showing me what it's like to break the rules. For inspiring and supporting me, always.

To Mr H. For being my partner in life and love. For your encouragement and support. For being my biggest (and often most challenging!) teacher.

To Mrs Baker. For 'publishing' my first story, The Wise Owl. For sparking my deep love of books and writing.

To Isobel Gatherer. For inspiring and encouraging me to just get it done and write this book! For being the channel for exactly what I needed to hear at the time.

To Jess Baker. For being my book buddy. For our weekly Skype chats and the immense power of accountability.

To Sam Richards-Hall. For being my pow wow partner. For providing an endlessly supportive space for me to grow and develop.

To Louise Lubke Cuss. For your amazing attention to detail and helping me to polish this manuscript.

To Lynda Mangoro. For your beautiful, intuitive designs. For just getting me (even when I'm finding it hard to explain what I want!).

To my clients and community. For your constant inspiration and support. For hearing me and being brave enough to be heard.

—

ABOUT THE AUTHOR

Nicola Humber is a hypnotherapist and coach, who specialises in helping women business-owners to make the income (and impact) they truly desire. She is passionate about helping her clients to move through any blocks and limitations so they can step into their full potential. ·

Since starting her hypnotherapy and coaching practice in 2010, Nicola has appeared on BBC Radio and written for publications, such as Natural Health magazine and Soul & Spirit.

At the time of writing Nicola lives on the south coast of England with her husband, Mark.

Contact Nicola

Find out more about Nicola and her work at www.nicolahumber.com.

You can also follow and connect with Nicola on social media:

www.facebook.com/nicolahumber

www.twitter.com/NicolaHumber

www.instagram.com/nicolahumber

Lightning Source UK Ltd.
Milton Keynes UK
UKHW050926290422
402257UK00006B/470